PACKAGING DRUGS
AND PHARMACEUTICALS

PACKAGING
DRUGS
AND
PHARMACEUTICALS

Wilmer A. Jenkins
Formerly Director
Packaging Products Division
Polymer Products Department
E. I. du Pont de Nemours & Company, Inc.

Kenton R. Osborn
Formerly Technology Manager
Packaging Products Division
Polymer Products Department
E. I. du Pont de Nemorus & Company, Inc.

CRC PRESS

Boca Raton   London   New York   Washington, D.C.

Library of Congress Cataloging-in-Publication Data

Main entry under title:
  Packaging Drugs and Pharmaceuticals.

Visit the CRC Press Web site at www.crcpress.com

© 1993 by CRC Press LLC

No claim to original U.S. Government works
International Standard Book Number 1-56676-014-3
Library of Congress Catalog Number 93-60377
Printed in the United States of America 1 2 3 4 5 6 7 8 9 0
Printed on acid-free paper

CONTENTS

PREFACE

Most people regard pharmaceuticals as vital life-preserving products that issue in a steady stream from a high technology industry whose scientific complexity puts it far beyond lay comprehension. They pay little attention to the packaging of these products except for spasms of annoyance at the impenetrable barrier the package occasionally erects between them and their medicine.

Yet the packaging of drugs is an activity nearly as important to the drug consumer as the manufacture of the drugs themselves. Without packages, essential medicines would never leave the drug factory. Without packages that protect pharmaceuticals from a hostile environment, product potency, purity and efficacy would all be compromised; the consequences to the patient could be fatal.

This book treats every facet of drug packaging in a comprehensive and highly readable way. It explains the *why* of drug packaging as well as the *what*, since a basic understanding of both what and why is the best foundation for comprehending any modern technology—and drug packaging is a technology more modern and complex than most people realize.

After beginning with a chapter which covers essential preliminary topics, the reader is then exposed in a systematic way to pharmaceutical dosage forms, the enormous regulatory umbrella that covers pharmaceutical packaging, the materials that are used to package drugs, the conversion of those materials into containers, the filling of the containers, the closures and the labels that complete the package, and finally, a description of how and why the various dosage forms and classes of drugs are packaged as they are. The last chapter examines three major issues that face today's drug packagers. A *Glossary* of terms and abbreviations can be found on pages 327–345.

The information in this book should be of value to many audiences:

- employees of companies that manufacture drugs, packages and packaging materials
- those working in pharmaceutical packaging who feel they need a broader comprehension of its many aspects as well as a reference source to keep them up to date
- pharmacy students and students pursuing a career in packaging

There is a small but significant difference in meaning between the words *drug* and *pharmaceutical*. A *drug* is generally taken to mean the active ingredient of the medicine; a *pharmaceutical* or *pharmaceutical product* is a manufactured article that often contains inactive ingredients which are aids to administration or which assist in the manufacturing process. Although it is *pharmaceuticals* and not *drugs* that are actually packaged, this book uses these terms as if they were synonymous; for reasons of brevity, "drug" is used more often than the more cumbersome "pharmaceutical."

ACKNOWLEDGEMENTS

As noted in the biographies, the authors have an extensive background in packaging, but when writing on any specialized topic, much detail must be gathered from current literature and from experts in the field. The authors welcome the opportunity to acknowledge here the assistance of a host of knowledgeable and cooperative individuals whose efforts have been essential to the completion of this work.

For helping us get organized in the field and develop a list of useful information sources, we thank John Moffett and Larry Hewlett, both formerly with Wyeth Laboratories; Dave Duerr, formerly with Richardson-Vick; Tom Savage of the Pharmaceutical Manufacturer's Association; Fred Simon of the Parenteral Drug Association; Bill Ellis of the Pennsylvania Society of Hospital Pharmacists; and Bill Bradley of the Non-Prescription Drug Manufacturer's Association.

Many people were willing to be interviewed, some several times and at great length. We thank them all for the invaluable information they provided: Tom Williams of PACO Corporation; Jeff Bourret, Director of the University of Pennsylvania Hospital Pharmacy; Bill Bradley of NPDMA; Knud Christiansen of Klockner-Pentaplast; Mike Cohen, Director of the Quakertown Community Hospital Pharmacy; Ed Hancock of American Mirrex; Dennis Kanemori of ICI Pharmaceuticals; Bob Miller of Fina Oil and Chemical Co.; Bruce and Ed Smith, both of the West Company; Kumar Nanavati of Sandoz Pharmaceuticals; Jim McTiernan of Hoffman La Roche; Gerald Frank of Rorer Pharmaceutical; Tom Ambrosio of Schering; Jim Komerska, a highly knowledgeable private consultant; and Larry Edzenga of SmithKline Beecham.

xi

The list of those who willingly supplied information to us over the telephone is a long one. Several FDA employees were most helpful: Barbara Ann Burke in Wilmington, DE, and Tony Lord and Paul Motise in Rockville, MD. Writers and editors of trade journals were an excellent information source: Frank Miele and Greg Lasoski at *Chain Drug Review*, Fred Rueckher at *Drugstore News*, Greg Erickson at *Packaging Magazine*, and Bob Heitzman at *Packaging Digest*.

Those with various associations not already acknowledged and whom we wish to thank for help are Stefanie Crawford of ASHP; John Cudahy and Laurie Root of IOPP; Ed Weary of the Flexible Packaging Association; Peter Mayberry and Dan Gerner at the Healthcare Packaging Council; Dave Prins, Bruce Siecker and Janet Scheren at the National Wholesale Drug Association; Meredith Scheck at the Vinyl Institute; Dorothy Smith of the Consumer Health Information Corporation; Andy Hait at the Bureau of the Census; Gordon Catto of the Proprietary Association of Great Britain; and Keith Johnson at USP.

As always, those in the business are one of the best information sources, and in that regard we are grateful for information gleaned from Bill Corbet of Huls America, Don Farrelly and Burton Spottiswoode of DuPont, Alan Johnston of Rexham Packaging, Andy Paul of the New Jersey Machine Company, Alexander Perritt of Perritt Laboratories, Bob Elcik of Occidental Chemicals, Jack Kirkpatrick of Sharp Packaging, and L. M. Hurst of the Association of the British Pharmaceutical Industry.

We are particularly grateful to the staffs of three excellent technical libraries in the Philadelphia area: the Lavoisier Library at the DuPont Experimental Station; the Joseph W. England Library at the Philadelphia College of Pharmacy and Science; and the Campbell Library at St. Joseph's University. The time that the always helpful and competent people in these organizations spent assisting us with information we needed was a major factor in the successful completion of this project.

And finally, our special thanks to packaging consultant Bob Kelsey, of Kelsey Corp., an editor and writer for *Food and Drug Packaging*, who reviewed the entire manuscript and made many helpful contributions.

CHAPTER ONE

Introduction

Healthcare in the U.S. is a huge and complex business, consuming $700 billion in expenditures that represent 13% of the gross national product [1]. Of this massive total, about 7%, or $50 billion, is spent on drugs for therapeutic purposes [2]. There are currently about 640 companies that manufacture drugs and pharmaceuticals, operating at 732 plant locations across the country [3]. The size of the drug packaging business is variously estimated at $3 to $4 billion with an annual growth rate of 9–10% [4].

This chapter presents the background material for the subsequent chapters that cover the various aspects of drug packaging. It begins by defining a drug and then moves to some general features of drug packaging followed by a section explaining the functions performed by a drug package. After sections that contrast drug packaging and food packaging and that describe the major trends in drug packaging, the size of the drug business and its principal components are discussed in more detail. The chapter concludes with a description of the various businesses that play a role in the creation, packaging and distribution of pharmaceutical products.

THE DEFINITION OF A DRUG

For this book, we have elected to use the definition used in the Federal Food, Drug, and Cosmetic Act of 1938 and later amended through 1989. That Act defines a drug as:

(A) articles recognized in the official United States Pharmacopoeia, Official Homeopathic Pharmacopoeia of the United

1

States, or Official National Formulary or any supplement to any of them;
(B) articles intended for use in the diagnosis, cure, mitigation, treatment, or prevention of disease in man or other animals; and
(C) articles (other than food) intended to affect the structure or any function of the body of man or other animals; and
(D) articles intended for use as a component of any articles specified in clause (A), (B), or (C); but does not include devices or their components, parts, or accessories. [5]

Medical devices, another huge business with its own set of packaging challenges, are not included in this book nor are other nontherapeutic products such as cosmetics, perfumes, and personal care items that dominate the shelves of most "drug" stores. We only deviate from this FDA Act definition by not treating animal drugs in a comprehensive way. As noted in the Preface, the terms *drug* and *pharmaceutical* are used as synonyms and only for variety; since *drug* is shorter, it appears more frequently.

GENERAL ASPECTS OF DRUG PACKAGING

The attitude of the general public towards the packaging of drugs, as compared to the product inside the package, may be best summed up by a quote from a national news daily [6]: "Packaging is an odd little corner of the drug business. It has a low public profile except in times of crisis." Most drug packaging engineers and the other professionals and companies involved in the packaging of drugs know differently: while it may have a low profile, it certainly isn't an "odd little corner." In fact, as this book will show, it is becoming an ever more important part of the total drug delivery system.

The Functions of a Drug Package

Containment

This is the most fundamental function of a drug package: to contain the packaged product and not allow it to become part of the environment. Principally, this requires a package that will not leak, that remains impervious to attack by the ingredients of drug formulations and that is strong enough to hold the contents during physical distribution.

Protection

After containment, protection is unquestionably the most important package function. The product must be protected against physical damage—such as breakage of tablets—against loss of contents or ingredients and against intrusion of unwanted components of the environment such as water vapor, oxygen, liquids, dirt and light.

Other Essential Functions

- The package must provide some way to dispense the contents, either into another container or directly onto the hand or into the body.
- Some provision must be made for reclosure of the package so the unused contents will not lose their potency or efficacy, become contaminated or represent a hazard to small children.
- When the package contents are sterile, this sterility must be maintained, including the sterility of the unused remainder.
- The package must present all the information about the drug that is required by law and good therapeutic practice.
- The package should help sell over-the-counter (OTC) products without the need for intervention by a pharmacist.
- Although most packages do not perform this function, packages which aid in compliance pay large dividends in reduced healthcare costs. This subject is developed more fully in Chapter Nine.
- The package design must provide evidence of tampering for those products which are so regulated by the FDA. Generally, all OTC drugs fall into this category.
- Packages for prescription drugs and certain OTC products must thwart access by young children.

DRUG PACKAGING VS.
FOOD PACKAGING

The technology required for packaging food is more varied and complex than is required by any other category of packaged goods. The packaging of drugs is a close second, well ahead of any other category of packaged products. These two packaging worlds have several package functions in common: containment, protection, identification and advertising of contents, need for ready access to contents and effective reclosability; but they differ in several interesting ways.

Many drugs can be harmful or even toxic unless taken in carefully regulated amounts. Although this is true of some foods as well, the "overdose" of any given food that is necessary to create a toxic effect is usually so large that other events (disinterest, nausea) occur before the overdose level is reached. This difference accounts for the child-resistant closures described in Chapter Six and the labeling requirements discussed in Chapter Seven.

Unless drugs are taken in the proper amounts and at the proper frequencies, they will be ineffective, and the patient's health may be at risk. Thus the *need for information to be conveyed* by the label is more crucial for drugs than for food and the *accuracy of the information* on the label is more important. The consequences of mislabeling foods are rarely fatal—mislabeled drugs are more likely to be lethal.

All food is taken into the body through the mouth, which is a nonsterile orifice. Thus the sterility requirements for foods and their packages are less stringent than they are for drugs that are, for example, injected directly into the bloodstream or into other subcutaneous regions of the body.

The alteration of the nature of a food product caused by improper choice of packaging materials is a serious matter, but drug/package interactions that alter the potency, sterility, or efficacy of a drug can have life-threatening consequences. These alterations may come about as a result of extraction of a package component by the drug, abstraction by the package material of a key component from the drug, reaction of atmospheric gases with the drug or by the action of light.

Unlike foods, almost all drugs look alike or, as in the case of aerosols, are packaged in opaque containers. Thus labeling which accurately describes the contents is crucial. For food products, on the other hand, the *billboard* or advertising functions of the package label are very important. This function is less important for drugs, which are often dispensed by pharmacists, doctors or nurses rather than being sold OTC.

Often, and particularly in the case of prescription drugs, the package contents are very expensive and the cost of the package is a much smaller fraction of the total product cost. This makes both the pressure and the incentive to reduce drug packaging costs less than the pressure to reduce food packaging costs.

Drugs are usually kept on the consumer's shelf far longer than are food products. This puts a special demand on the package design to protect the contents against slow deterioration and on the package label to convey a realistic expiration date.

The packaging of drugs is more tightly regulated than is the packaging of foods. For example, the U.S. Pharmacopoeia (USP) recommends package types for over 1500 pharmaceutical products. These recommendations have the force of law. No such situation exists for food products. One consequence of this highly regulated atmosphere is that drug packages, as compared to food packages, are slow to change.

Point-of-sale repackaging is uncommon for food products but very common in drug packaging. The unit dose concept that is gradually taking hold will make repackaging by the pharmacist less common, as will the trend towards offering more drugs OTC.

Tamper evidence is regarded as more crucial for drugs than for food. There is no logic to this, since food is also tampered with, but no regulations exist for food like those for drugs, largely because food packaging is so huge and varied that self-regulation is the only practical course and because the tighter profit margins on food make the addition of tamper evident features to food packages a more consequential cost factor.

The necessity to make packages friendly for the elderly is a bigger issue for drugs than for food. There are several reasons for this:

- Drug consumption is skewed towards the elderly.
- Medication is probably more vital to the survival of the elderly than to the younger segment of the population.
- Elderly people rarely have to cook for the young but the reverse is not true; thus a disproportionate share of food packages are handled by younger people.

- Compliance is not an issue with food products, but is a growing issue with drugs and is partly a drug packaging issue.

MAJOR TRENDS IN DRUGS THAT AFFECT PACKAGING

Over-the-Counter Distribution

The growing cost of healthcare and the marketing thrust of some drug companies both lead to an increasing number of drug products being offered over the counter. Although six of every ten medications purchased in 1988 were bought OTC, only two cents of the healthcare dollar is spent on OTC drugs. A typical U.S. patient spends $16 for a prescription drug as against $4 for an OTC drug [7]. In 1987, $24 billion in healthcare costs was saved by the use of OTC medications [8] and it has been estimated that by the year 2000, the savings will grow to $34 billion [9].

There are other reasons for the trend towards OTC marketing of drugs:

- OTC drugs will successfully cure or ameliorate some unpleasant symptoms. It is simpler to self-medicate than put up with the inconvenience and expense of seeing a doctor.
- There are additional profits to be made. Not all prescription-to-OTC switches have been successful, but it is not uncommon for a company to increase sales fivefold for a product after making it available OTC [10].
- The exclusivity once enjoyed by many prescription drugs has been eroded in recent years by the growth of generic equivalents. These now exceed $5 billion in volume [11] and represent one-third of all the prescriptions filled [12]. Generic equivalents often appear soon after patent protection expires, causing the original producer's profits to drop sharply. In that event, the OTC market offers possibilities for recouping part of those losses through increased sales volume.
- The aging population guarantees a greater market for drugs of all kinds. Not only is the overall market increasing, but

the elderly, who can spend more time and give more
thought to taking care of themselves, are more likely to
favor OTC drugs because of their lower cost and the
opportunity they offer to be independent of a doctor.

The near-term annual growth in the OTC market, estimated at
greater than 9% [12], will be fueled by at least 50 petitions to the
FDA for switches planned in the next five years [13] and by the
switching of several classes of drugs: three nonsedating antihistamines for allergy/sinus/cold relief; five nonsteroidal anti-inflammatory drugs as improved analgesics; several ulcer medications; a
new class of antifungal drugs to treat gynecological yeast infections; muscle relaxants; products to treat skin and eye irritations;
gum formulated to discourage smoking; and Rogaine, to cure
baldness. The move of these products to OTC will increase the
dollar volume of all OTC products by 40% [10].

Switching drugs to the OTC market has a major impact on drug
packaging. The sober, functional, sterile-looking package used for
delivery of product to pharmacist and hospital must be replaced
by a package which stresses brand name and uses color to distinguish the product from its competition. The package must effectively advertise the product and clearly state what it does for the
customer in addition to providing clear instructions for how to
use and not misuse the medication. Although the package appearance must be more dramatic, the manufacturer must be careful not to overdo it—credibility and the image of responsibility
and safety must be retained [14].

The information that must be conveyed to the consumer on OTC
drug packages is voluminous—far greater than for any other category of packaged products. For example, it must include the manufacturer's name; the brand name; the use for which the product
is intended; the quantity of product contained within the package; a prominent statement that explains what tamper evident
feature has been incorporated; instructions and warnings connected with use; the beneficial results that should follow the use
of the product; information, if any, which sets this product apart
from competitive offerings; expiration date information, if applicable; information on how the product must be stored if the
contents are sensitive to heat or light.

An additional complication of OTC switching arises when
retail establishments that do not employ a pharmacist sell OTC

drugs. In such cases, the consumer's only information source is the label. This puts additional demands on label design and content, two areas of drug packaging that are being increasingly criticized.

We will discuss labeling requirements and problems in detail in Chapter Seven. The point made here is that the major package redesign necessitated by an OTC switch qualifies the OTC trend as *the* major trend influencing drug packaging today.

Liquids to Solids

In the early years of the 20th century, available medications were frequently unpleasant tasting liquids. Later developments have shifted the product balance to solids which can be swallowed rapidly with no unpleasant taste sensation. Thus over 70% of all oral medications are now solids. This trend has far-reaching packaging implications. Its greatest single beneficiary is the blister package discussed in Chapter Five.

Unit Dose Packaging

A complete discussion of unit dose packaging and the many issues it involves is presented in Chapter Nine, and is simply mentioned here since it is a major drug trend with a strong influence on packaging.

Administration Aids

As discussed in Chapters Six and Eight, packages are becoming more consumer friendly. For example, they now contain devices which put the drug where it should go and in the right amount: plastic squeeze bottles, droppers, transdermal delivery systems, prefilled syringes, droppers, and pump and aerosol sprays.

The Aging Population

The elderly population in the U.S. is growing at 2% per year, twice the rate of growth of the overall population. In addition, the elderly segment is aging, with a steadily larger proportion reaching seventy-five years old or older [15]. These trends have a major influence on the drug business and drug packaging. The elderly

20% of the population accounts for 50% of the healthcare costs and consumes a disproportionate share of all pharmaceutical preparations [16]. This is the major reason for the growth in pharmaceutical sales being more than twice the growth in sales of all other manufactured products. Package design continues to reflect this key demographic trend in myriad ways ranging from design changes for the OTC market favored by the elderly to changes in child-resistant closure regulations intended to make life easier for the infirm.

THE SIZE OF THE DRUG BUSINESS IN THE U.S.

Overall Sales

In terms of retail dollar sales, the drug business *as we have defined it* totaled $49.3 billion in 1990 [17]. This figure does *not* include the closely related field of personal care products nor does it include nontherapeutic product categories such as baby products, contraceptive preparations, vitamins, diet aids, nutritional supplements, feminine hygiene products, contact lens preparations, denture adhesives and cleaners, and so forth.

The major categories that make up this total are:

- prescription drugs: $36 billion
- OTC drugs: $8.4 billion
- hospitals: $5 billion

Since these are dollar figures, they do not accurately reflect the physical volume sold. Various estimates [18] suggest that the physical volume split between OTC and prescription drugs is about 60–40 in favor of OTC.

Sales by Product Category

Table 1.1 shows how sales of prescription drugs are divided among the major drug categories. Although the latest available data are for the year 1986, they are still of interest [19].

The best comparable data for OTC drugs are shown in Table 1.2 [20]. They are more recent (1990) but are limited to sales in chain drugstores. Since chains account for about 50% of total retail drug

Table 1.1. *Sales of prescription drugs by product category.*

Category	% of Total Dollar Sales Volume
Central Nervous System	24.7
Cardiovascular	19.6
Anti-Infectives	16.9
Neoplasms and Endocrine	13.0
Gastrointestinal and Genitourinary	11.2
Respiratory System	6.3
Vitamins and Nutrients	3.8
Dermatologicals	2.3
All Other	2.3

outlet sales, we may take these as reasonably representative of the $8.4 billion total.

There are interesting trends in the analgesics market that do not appear in the figures in Table 1.2 [20]:

- Aspirin's share of the analgesic market fell about 4 points to 39.5% in spite of studies suggesting its benefits in preventing heart attacks.

Table 1.2. *Sales of OTC drugs by product category.*

Category	% of Total Dollar Sales Volume*
Cough/Cold	
Solids	10.3
Liquids	6.6
Analgesics	12.3
Dental Care	10.1
Laxatives	5.5
Antacids	5.2
First Aid	5.1
Footcare	3.5
Antidiarrhea/Antinausea	1.5
Acne	1.5
Sleeping Aids	0.6
Asthma Preparations	0.3

*These figures do not add up to 100% since we have not included some large product categories such as nutritional supplements which do not fall within our definition of a drug.

- Ibuprofen's share (21%) increased at the expense of acetaminophen (38%) as Advil and Motrin IB gained in popularity due to their anti-inflammatory features.
- Another nighttime analgesic containing acetaminophen plus a sleep-inducing component was introduced.

Relationship to Other Industries

Compared to other major industries in the U.S., the pharmaceutical manufacturing industry is not particularly large in dollar sales, ranking below the first five companies on the Fortune 500 list, but by the standards of the giants, it is impressively profitable. In 1987 for example, after-tax earnings as a percent of sales were 10.5% compared to 4.9% for all manufacturing [21].

THE DRUG PACKAGING BUSINESS

This section will cover the spectrum of participants in drug packaging: drug manufacturers, contract packagers, repackagers, package and packaging material manufacturers, hospitals and pharmacists in retail drug outlets. For this material to make sense, however, we must first deal in a preliminary way with the materials and the types of packages that are used.

Materials

U.S. drug packagers spend an estimated $3 billion on drug packages and packaging materials, and about six billion rigid containers were consumed by pharmaceutical packagers in 1990. Plastic packages now have about 80% of this market which consumes about $200 million worth of plastic resins [22]. Glass and metal, once the dominant materials, have long been losing share to plastic. Some authorities predict that glass and metal consumption will decline in absolute terms while others believe that the overall market growth at 9% will lead to some growth in these traditional materials as well [23]. OTC products have provided the largest opportunity for plastics' growth, but since this market is now largely converted to plastics, liquid drugs for hospitals and unit dose blister packages will be the future growth areas for plastics. The lightweight, easy storage, shatterproof and fabrication flexibility features of plastics are quite important in these two applications.

As noted below, bottles and vials are the most common pharmaceutical containers. Table 1.3 gives a breakdown of the 1990 usage of various plastic materials in this application.

The pharmaceutical closure market is also dominated by plastic. Table 1.4 gives the breakdown for 1990.

Package Types

Table 1.5 shows the frequency of use in 1991 of different drug packages, expressed as a percentage of the total dollars spent on all types [24].

Participants

Drug Manufacturers

The latest count [3] shows 640 drug manufacturers in the U.S. The prescription drug industry is only modestly concentrated. In 1982, the four largest companies accounted for about one-fourth of the total shipments and it took over twenty companies to account for 70% of total shipments [25]. The OTC segment has about the same concentration; about ten companies control almost 50% of the business [26].

The primary function of these companies is to develop, manufacture and sell pharmaceuticals for humans and animals. Thus they concentrate on research which creates new products, on improving manufacturing techniques to lower cost and improve quality, and on more effective marketing of their products. In these activities, packaging has always been recognized as a necessary function, but not a central one. In fact, many drug companies still use contract packagers to an important degree. It is estimated that 15% of all drugs manufactured in the U.S. are packaged by contract packagers [27].

This view of packaging has been changing over the last one or two decades, as companies face the issues and opportunities that focus on packaging, of which the following are a sample:

- the trend to OTC marketing
- continuing problems with mislabeling

Table 1.3. Plastics volume in pharmaceutical bottles and vials [24].

Resin	Volume (million lbs)
HDPE	208
LDPE and LLDPE	26
PET	26
PP	26
PS	10
PVC	26
Total	310

Table 1.4. Plastics volume in pharmaceutical closures [24].

Resin	Volume (million lbs)
PP	52
PS	21
HDPE	12
PVC	5
LDPE	4
Total	94

Table 1.5. Frequency of use of various containers.

Container	% of Total 1991 Dollar Sales
Plastic Containers	24.7
Paperboard Containers	21.3
Blister Packages	11.9
Labels and Package Inserts	11.1
Plastic Closures	10.8
Glass Containers	7.1
Metal Containers	4.0
Nonplastic Closures	3.4
Miscellaneous	5.7

- the persistent tampering problem
- the opportunities for design innovation offered by plastics
- the heightened emphasis on cost reduction brought about by greater foreign competition

The large drug companies now have package engineering departments that are responsible for:

- developing packaging for new products
- ensuring lowest cost raw materials by developing a stable of qualified vendors
- reducing costs of packaging by looking broadly at the entire manufacturing and marketing operations and their impact on package costs
- optimizing packaging and the packaging process for existing products
- giving technical support to packaging operations

The pharmaceutical industry is composed of individual manufacturers who differ from each other but who have a few characteristics in common. They see their future profitability depending on developing differentiated products that can be kept exclusive for a time through patents. Thus they tend to be highly research oriented, spending over 10% of their sales dollars on R&D [28]. Towards functions like packaging, they are slow to change as compared to food companies. This conservatism is not inherent in the personalities of the company managers—rather it is the result of the complex, expensive, time-consuming approval process required by the FDA before a drug package can be changed. In contrast to food companies, the rate of new drug product introduction is orders of magnitude slower and is usually not linked to the introduction of a new package to accompany the drug. Finally, since drug companies rely on the package to help differentiate and sell their products only in the OTC market, the overall reliance on the sales effect of the package is less than for food companies.

Contract Packagers

There are 330 companies in the U.S. whose function is the packaging of products manufactured by others [29]. Of these, less than 10% package drugs, largely because of the myriad special requirements and regulations that surround that activity.

Contract packagers are highly skilled in packaging operations, have a variety of packaging machines available for a diversity of packaging jobs, employ package designers to help the manufacturer choose the style and type of package and specialize in making short runs as compared to the long runs favored by the product manufacturer whose diversity of packaging skills and equipment are often limited.

Drug companies use contract packagers in several different situations:

- when introducing a new OTC product where the manufacturer wants to market test several different package designs
- during the sampling of a product before full-scale introduction
- in the development of a new package, when the manufacturer wants to experiment with a variety of package types and designs
- in the early part of a product's life cycle when the volume is small

All these situations have one element in common: the number of items packaged is relatively small. Contract packagers can make short runs more readily than the drug companies can.

However, not all the contract packager's business is limited to temporary situations and short runs. As noted above, about 15% of the U.S. drug volume is contract packaged on an ongoing basis for drug companies who prefer to invest their effort and capital in other essential functions.

The successful contract packager is innovative, flexible, and service oriented. Many are the first to purchase the latest models of packaging machinery so they can introduce new packaging techniques to their clients. In these ways, they attempt to differentiate themselves from their competition and remain on the leading edge of new packaging developments and techniques. Many of the drug packages that are now common were codesigned by contract packagers.

Contract drug packagers are governed by the same set of "Current Good Manufacturing Practices" (CGMP) requirements (see Chapter Three) that apply to the operations of the drug manufacturers.

Drug Repackagers

In contrast to contract packaging, drug repackaging is an operation set up to supply hospitals, group practitioners, and physicians with consumer-sized quantities of drugs in packages that enable them to dispense these prescription drugs in unit dose form directly to the patient without any further repackaging.

Repackaging is a relatively small business with few participants. Volume numbers are difficult to obtain because some contract packagers also perform this function. Companies that only repackage had about $25 million in sales in 1987, but it was then projected, probably optimistically, that their business would grow by 1992 to $1 or $2 billion, still less than 5% of total drug sales [30]. The growth of this segment of the drug packaging business will depend largely on the growth of direct physician dispensing, a complex issue with many legal and political ramifications that are outside the scope of this book [31].

MANUFACTURERS OF DRUG PACKAGES AND PACKAGING MATERIALS

The Flexible Packaging Converter

Manufacturers of flexible plastic packages are called converters. A typical converter buys raw materials such as plastic resins and films, adhesives, inks, paper and aluminum foil and combines them on the converting machinery described in Chapters Four and Five to produce flexible packages such as pouches or blister packs. The converter also makes rolls of printed film that are sold to a packager who creates a package and fills it with his product in a single operation. Creation of the package by the product manufacturer in this way is common in the food industry but rare in pharmaceutical packaging operations.

The film sold by converters usually consists of several layers. Since most flexible drug packages consist of only one layer of film, drug manufacturers often buy film directly from the film manufacturers and some even make their own film from purchased resins. Thus the *flexible* packaging converters play a minor role in the drug packaging chain compared to the major role they play in the food packaging chain. The fundamental reason for this lies in the difference between flexible drug packages and flexible food packages; the latter are more complex structures and generally carry far more elaborate graphics than do flexible drug packages. The flexible packaging converter is successful because of expertise in creating complex structures and elaborate graphics. Since food manufacturers need these products far more than drug companies, the converter concentrates his efforts on the food packaging market.

The Rigid Packaging Converter

The traditional rigid plastic packages which are very common in drug packaging are never made by the drug manufacturer but always by a rigid packaging converter. This situation is analogous to the role played by the manufacturers of rigid glass and metal containers for drugs, which are always manufactured either by the companies that make the raw materials or by companies specially created for the purpose. Thus when plastic bottles and jars appeared, it was natural for the drug companies to depend on some other company to make these as well. This dependence was encouraged by glass container manufacturers who wanted to become the dominant suppliers of plastic containers as well.

DISTRIBUTORS OF PACKAGED DRUGS

Drug wholesalers play an important role in the flow of drugs from manufacturer to final consumer: about 75% of drug manufacturer's sales of prescription drugs are to wholesalers, with the balance split about evenly between retailers and hospitals [32]. Wholesalers' customers for prescription drugs are:

- independent drug stores — 41%
- chain drug stores — 22%
- hospitals — 24%

- mass marketers — 3%
- other wholesalers — 8%
- other — 2%

Thus two-thirds of prescription drugs flow to the consumer via retail drug outlets and one-third flows via hospitals. Adding to these figures the OTC volume, which is all sold in retail outlets, we conclude that the more than 40,000 retail outlets handle about 75% of all drug sales to consumers. The nation's 6700 hospitals account for about 15%, mail order sales about 6%, and sales by physicians the remainder. It is estimated [33] that 15% of primary care physicians now dispense prescription drugs.

This final stage of distribution includes repackaging of prescription drugs in both hospitals and retail pharmacies. Many hospitals now repackage their solid dosage forms for internal dispensing rather than having the floor nurse pour out the correct dose from a bulk container into a small paper cup. Blister and strip packs are the principal package forms used by hospitals for repackaging solids. This means that hospital pharmacists must buy film and other components and operate blister and strip packaging equipment, even though such an operation should be performed by a packaging professional. Retail pharmacists repackage most of the solid and liquid dosage forms they sell. The involvement in repackaging by hospital and retail pharmacists is a direct consequence of the minor role played by unit dose packaging by manufacturers in the U.S. We will return to this subject in Chapter Nine where the status and future of unit dose packaging are examined in some detail.

REFERENCES

1. Hilts, P. J. 1991. *New York Times* (May 19): section 4, p. 1.
2. Anon. 1991. *Drugstore News* (April 22):17; Anon. 1988. *PMA Statistical Facts*, p. 3.
3. Andrew Hait, Bureau of the Census, private communication, June 5, 1991.
4. Anon. 1988. *Packaging Digest* (August):8; Anon. 1991. *Paper, Film, and Foil Converter* (August):10.
5. Federal Food, Drug and Cosmetic Act, Sect. 201 (U.S. Code Title 21, Section 321), Chapter 2 — Definitions.
6. Markiewicz, D. 1991. *USA Today* (March 25).

7. Anon. 1991. *Packaging Digest* (September):6.

8. *U.S. Industrial Outlook 1989*, p. 16-3.

9. Anon. 1988. *Packaging Digest* (August):8.

10. Anon. 1991. *Drug Topics* (May 20):36.

11. *U.S. Industrial Outlook 1989*, p. 16-4.

12. Blyth, J. S. 1991. *Pharm. Exec.* (March):86.

13. Anon. 1991. *Chain Drug Review* (January 1).

14. Blyth, J. S. 1982. *Pharm. Exec.* (March):48.

15. Anon. 1991. *N.Y. Times* (March 10):E4.

16. *U.S. Industrial Outlook 1989*, p. 16-1.

17. Anon. 1991. *Drugstore News* (April 22):20; Anon. 1988. *PMA Statistical Facts*, p. 6; private communications from various industry sources.

18. Anon. 1988. *Packaging Digest* (August):8; private communications from various industry sources.

19. Anon. 1988. *PMA Statistical Facts*, p. 4.

20. Anon. 1991. *Drugstore News* (April 22):20.

21. Anon. 1988. *PMA Statistical Facts*, p. 19.

22. Anon. 1991. In Frost and Sullivan, *The U.S. Market for Plastic Materials Used in Pharmaceutical and Medical Applications*, A2378 (April); Hess. 1992. *Proceedings of Conference on Pharmaceutical Packaging Outlook '92*, Avalon Communications, P.O. Box 505, Southampton, PA 18966.

23. Anon. 1991. *Paper Film and Foil Converter* (August):10.

24. Martineau, W. D. and J. C. Forman. 1992. *Proceedings of Conference on Pharmaceutical Packaging Outlook '92*, Avalon Communications, P.O. Box 505, Southampton, PA 18966.

25. Anon. 1988. *PMA Statistical Facts*, p. 14.

26. *U.S. Industrial Outlook 1987*, p. 16-4.

27. T. Williams, PACO Corp., private communication, April, 1992.

28. *U.S. Industrial Outlook 1989*, p. 16-1.

29. 1989. *IOPP Directory of Contract Packagers and Their Facilities*, 2nd Edition.

30. Anon. 1987. *American Druggist* (September):62.

31. Anon. 1987. *Packaging Digest* (May):26.

32. Anon. 1988. *PMA Statistical Facts*, p. 5; National Wholesale Drug Association, private communication, May, 1991.

33. *U.S. Industrial Outlook 1989*, p. 16-3.

CHAPTER TWO

Drugs and Pharmaceuticals and Their Various Dosage Forms

The purpose of this chapter is to provide a fundamental understanding of those characteristics of drugs, pharmaceuticals and dosage forms which determine packaging needs. To this end, four topics which are important for all drugs and dosage forms are covered first: stability, purity, sterility and drug physiology. With this understanding in place, descriptions of the various dosage forms and their packaging needs come next.

STABILITY

The first consideration in the formulation of a drug product is to provide effective and safe treatment of specific medical conditions. A close second is the concern that the medication maintain its effectiveness from the time of manufacture to the moment of use. Assurance of effectiveness requires the absence of both physical and chemical change. Physical changes (e.g., the settling out of a suspension or the breakup of a tablet) in a drug product will be dealt with in later sections where the various dosage forms are described. Here only chemical reactions are considered.

Most drugs are complex organic molecules and their biological activity depends not only on the specific constituents but often on the exact configuration of these constituents within the molecule. Optical isomers, for example, are forms of a molecule that differ only by the change in position by rotation of some chemical group around a central carbon atom. Often one form (the l or levo form) is more pharmaceutically active than the other (the d or dextro form). Thus, l-epinephrine is 15–20 times more active in treating severe allergic reactions than the d form.* The structures for these two optical isomers are shown in Figure 2.1. Transformations of optical isomers can be triggered by mild heat or light. This susceptibility to chemical change under fairly mild conditions is not uncommon for drugs, since to be biologically active generally means they must be chemically reactive.

Since very subtle chemical changes can markedly change a drug's potency, detection of such alteration is frequently difficult. Sometimes changes related to potency reduction such as discoloration or precipitate formation in a solution can be observed. A direct measure of potency is obtained from in vivo tests (that is, tests in humans or animals) but these are time-consuming and expensive. Therefore, quantitative assay techniques, often very sophisticated and specific to a given drug, are developed to measure the concentration of the active components. In general, 90% retention of potency is the minimum acceptable level. This level is the end point on which expiration dates are normally based. Beyond loss of drug potency is the additional possibility of building up harmful by-products from continuing chemical reactions in the drug formulation. Fortunately, incidents of this kind have been rare.

Some compounds or mixtures are inherently unstable. It is the task of the pharmaceutical manufacturer and pharmacist to develop formulations and processing conditions to overcome this instability. In many cases, however, this chemical instability is initiated or accelerated by factors in the environment such as heat and light. The package can have significant impact on some, but not all, of these factors. For example, the package cannot give long term protection against heat. At best, insulating materials such as foams can be used to protect from short term thermal shocks. Thus, the discussion that follows will focus on drug degradation processes that are affected by moisture, oxygen and light.

Moisture

Many pharmaceuticals contain ester or amide functional groups which can react with water, leading to the cleavage of a chemical bond and the creation of two new species. For drugs

---

*Whenever a generic or chemical name of a drug first appears in this chapter and
Chapter Eight, the product category or use will be given.

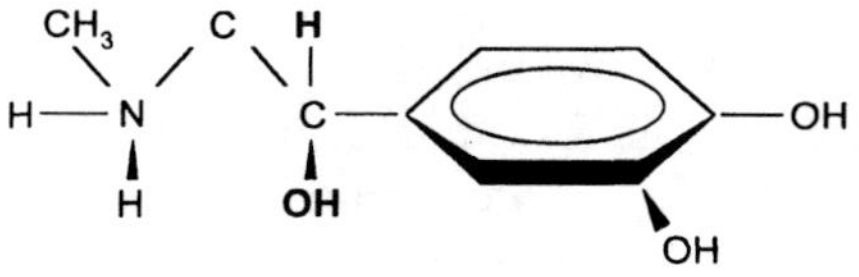

FIGURE 2.1. The molecular structures of *d*- and *l*-epinephrine.

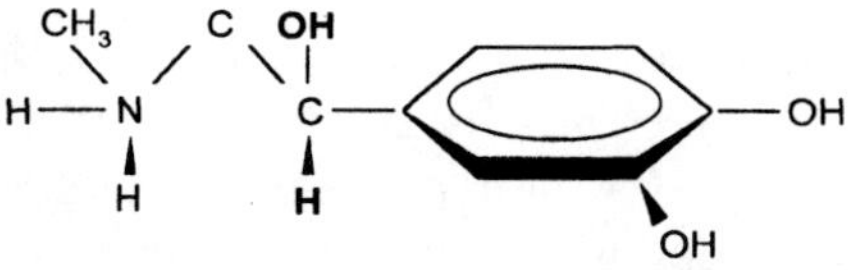

with an ester group the new products are an acid and an alcohol; for an amide group an acid and an amine are formed. These reactions are shown in Figure 2.2. Specific drugs prone to hydrolysis include aspirin; cocaine, procaine, and tetracaine (anesthetics); physostigmine (used to counteract central nervous system drugs); atropine (used to increase heart rate); thiamine and niacinamide (nutritional supplements); and phenethicillin and benzylpenicillin (antibiotics).

While hydrolysis can occur in pure water, generally a catalyst is required for initiation. Both acids and bases are catalysts but basic conditions are usually more effective. For drug solutions, optimization and control of pH by the addition of small amounts of acid or base or buffering agents can minimize this kind of hydrolysis. Reducing the concentration of water by adding alternate sol-

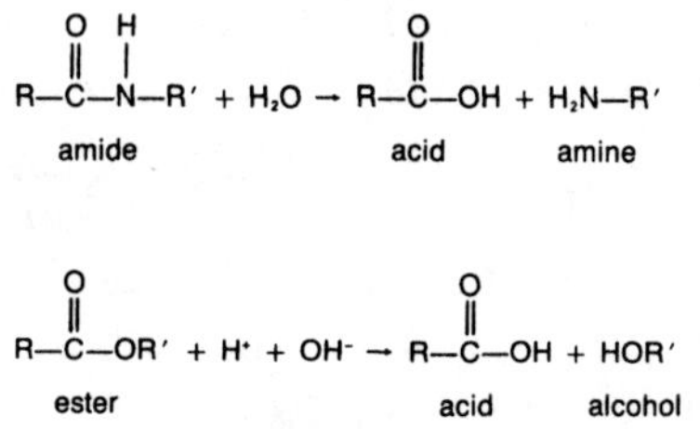

FIGURE 2.2. The hydrolysis of amides and esters.

vents can also help. For example, barbiturates are much more stable in propylene glycol–water mixtures than in pure water. Surfactants reduce hydrolysis by shielding the susceptible groups from the attacking ions. In this way the half-life of benzocaine, an anesthetic, can be increased by a factor of 18.

Oxygen

Many drugs are adversely affected by oxygen: steroids, vitamins, antibiotics and epinephrine. The oxidation process involves the removal of electrons from an atom and may not require the presence of oxygen. When oxygen is involved, often only small amounts are needed to set off a chain reaction propagated by free radicals. Oxidation reactions can be inhibited by antioxidants and free radical scavengers. In aqueous systems these inhibitors include sulfites, thiosulfates, and ascorbic acid, while for oil-based systems ascorbyl palmitate, hydroquinone, propyl gallate, and nordihydroguaiaretic acid are effective. Since the last traces of oxygen are difficult to remove, packages are sometimes flushed with inert gases, such as nitrogen or carbon dioxide. In some cases, oxidation is catalyzed by heavy metals and hydronium and hydroxyl ions so that eliminating or neutralizing these is also effective. Drugs that are susceptible to oxidation, especially in the presence of heavy metals, include penicillin, epinephrine, phenylephrine (a decongestant), lincomycin (an antibiotic), isoprenaline and procaine hydrochloride.

Light

When an organic molecule absorbs light it is activated to a higher energy level. The extent of this activation depends on the wavelength of light. Ultraviolet light, being more energetic, is much more effective than visible light and provides enough energy to rupture a chemical bond to form free radicals. Often oxidation is photochemically initiated in this manner if both light and oxygen are present. Sometimes molecules that are photo-activated do not themselves undergo chemical reaction but transfer their energy upon collision with other molecules. Also racemization, the change from one optical isomer to another which was described above, is often caused by the absorption of light. Examples of drugs that undergo simple chemical bond cleavage in the presence of light are chlorpromazine (used to treat psychotic disorders); and hydrocortisone, prednisolone, and methylprednisolone (steroids). Since degradation occurs by free radical processes, antioxidants can be effective inhibitors.

Prediction of Shelf Life

The kinetics of degradation of many drugs have been elucidated leading to mathematical equations from which shelf life (usually the point in time when potency reaches 90% of the labeled value) can be predicted fairly accurately. On the other hand it is not necessary to determine the mechanism of the reaction for predictive purposes. As long as an assay method can be used to measure either the concentration of the drug or its degraded form versus time, then the data can be linearized by some empirical mathematical approach and extrapolated with good confidence. The shape of the curves of product loss versus time are not very dependent on the mechanism for a loss of less than 50%. Statistical techniques and computer modeling greatly simplify and speed up the extrapolation. Often data are obtained over several temperatures for added confidence in the determination of shelf life. While fairly crude data may be sufficient for guidance during product optimization, shelf life data on a product ready to market is usually extensive and includes samples from a number of production lots. Finally, to compensate for potency loss due to instability, initial drug content is typically higher than the labeled amount. It is recommended that this overage be no more than 30%.

Packaging Needs

For moisture and oxygen sensitive drugs, protection from these substances is required. However, with inhibitors in the formulation and the use of overage, it is relatively rare that complete elimination of oxygen and moisture is necessary. There is also a need to avoid the introduction of substances, such as heavy metals, that could act as catalysts and that could come from the environment or the package. For light sensitive drugs, complete elimination of light, especially the ultraviolet wavelengths, is essential. Again, there is the need to avoid trace contaminants that could act as photoinitiators. Finally, it is important that additives critical to product stability, such as antioxidants, not interact with the package.

PURITY AND STERILITY

Purity and sterility are required attributes of commercial pharmaceuticals and are achieved primarily by the diligent application of well established technology day in and day out during the manufacture of the product. Assuming a drug has been formulated to achieve the effectiveness and safety claimed, then the total manufacturing operation must be designed and controlled to assure that product variability and all forms of biological and chemical contamination are kept within acceptable limits. Guidelines for achieving these objectives are now part of the regulations set forth by the FDA and are published under the title: Current Good Manufacturing Practice in Manufacture, Processing, Packing or Holding Human and Veterinary Drugs [1].

Thus the drug industry is infused with a strong quality control emphasis that includes continual checking for approval or rejection of raw materials, packaging components and product (in-process as well as finished product); inspection of all stages of the operation; and extensive record keeping. These activities are carried out by a separate, dedicated department as part of the total quality program in which every member of the manufacturing organization is dedicated to achieving assurance of product quality. Further quality assurance is achieved by the validation procedures described in Chapter Three.

Given this general picture of the approaches to assure drug quality, the specific problem of microbial contamination must now be discussed. This can be an even more serious problem than drug stability, especially for the manufacturer of liquid products. In recent years, microbial contamination has led to recalls of products as diverse as baby lotion and milk of magnesia. Tests on retail packages of antacid preparations revealed that 30.5% of the bottles contained *Pseudomonas aeruginosa* with aerobic plate counts as high as 93,000 organisms per gram. The microorganisms identified in other instances include *Salmonella sp.*, *E. coli*, certain *Pseudomonas sp.* and *Staphylococcus aureus*. [2].

Liquids can be ideal growth media for bacteria as can be many of the raw materials, especially natural products, used in their preparation. Bacteria also flourish in the difficult-to-clean parts of processing equipment. Thus monitoring of materials and thorough cleaning are essential. Furthermore, the atmosphere in manufacturing operations needs to be monitored to assure that a maximum level of microbial contamination is not being exceeded. Microbial monitoring of process water is also essential.

Routine testing is recommended for bacteria in some classes of finished products such as oral solutions and suspensions for *E. coli*, topical preparations for *P. aeruginosa* and *S. aureus* and products for rectal, urethral, or vaginal administration for total bacterial count. In addition to these operational procedures, antibacterial preservatives are often used in liquid preparations and are almost mandatory for water containing products. Common preservatives are alcohols, phenol, hexachlorophene, mercury compounds, and benzoic acids and esters. Some of these are restricted from oral preparations.

While the problem of bacterial contamination of so-called nonsterile drug preparations has received recent reemphasis, sterile drug products, such as those intended for ophthalmic or parenteral use, have always been subject to stringent requirements. The possibility that contaminated drug preparations could cause serious ocular infection has been well documented. One bacillus, *Pseudomonas aeruginosa*, is especially virulent since it grows readily in ophthalmic solutions and can cause blindness in 24 to 48 hours. While the most likely source of contamination is from reuse of containers or droppers that have contacted infected areas, contamination has been found in freshly dispensed solutions, typically with the most common bacillus, the staphylococcus group. Antimicrobial additives help but are not foolproof since, for example, viruses are not affected.

The preferred route to insuring product sterility is terminal sterilization: processing the finished, packaged product under conditions that will deactivate microbes. The most common method is to use steam or dry heat. Alternatives include high and low energy radiation and gases.

Another approach is aseptic filling. Here the product and the package are separately sterilized and brought together in an aseptic environment. The areas where parenteral drugs are handled and filled into sterile containers are generally *Class 100* areas, which means that there must be per cubic foot of air less than 100 particles 0.5 microns in size or larger. This is achieved by air filtration, scrupulous cleanliness, and constant monitoring.

Another contaminant of concern is pyrogens which are substances that induce fever, especially when administered by injection. While there are many pyrogens, endotoxin, a residue from
gram-negative bacteria, is the most important one in sterile drug
manufacture. Pyrogens can be present in crude drugs such as antibiotics, or in water, or they can come from contamination during
processing. Purification steps usually take care of raw materials as
a source of pyrogens. Stringent procedures during manufacture
will eliminate in-process contamination. Depyrogenation of surfaces is achieved by heating at 250°C for 45 minutes or by heating
in the presence of alkali or strong oxidizing solutions. Thorough
washing with detergent is also claimed to be effective. Careful
protection of cleaned surfaces is essential.

Packaging Needs

Within the environment of total quality control in the manufacture of pharmaceuticals, packaging must consistently meet
agreed-upon specifications such as level of protection. It is also
critical that packaging not be a source of contamination. Where
sterilization of the package or packaged drug product is part of the
manufacturing process, the packaging material must withstand
these forms of sterilization. For aseptic filling, the package must
be produced and stored under conditions that preserve sterility.

DRUG PHYSIOLOGY

When drug therapy is administered topically for localized effect
only, the physiology is relatively straightforward, since the drug
is put in direct contact with the condition to be treated such as a
burned area, a laceration or athlete's foot. On the other hand,
where therapy requires introduction of the drug into the circulatory system to achieve a systemic effect, as in the use of an antibiotic to treat an infection, the situation is much more complicated.

Several routes are used to achieve systemic access. The most
direct is injection into a vein or artery as in the administration of
intravenous fluids. Introduction into the bloodstream can be
delayed and distributed over a longer period of time by injection,
for instance, into muscle tissue. Ingestion of drugs via the gas-

trointestinal tract using tablets or liquids is a more indirect route. Finally, there is the introduction through the skin and mucous membranes where medications must be absorbed from ointments, liquids, mists or patches. Each of these access routes involves different physiology.

The Injection Route

The injection route has the advantage of directness. Therapeutic benefits are quicker. Control is better since the irregularities of intestinal absorption are avoided. Administration can be achieved even when the patient is unwilling or unable to swallow. On the other hand, antiseptic conditions are required for administration, there can be local tissue irritation, and introduction into the bloodstream of contaminants or incorrect dosages is swift and sometimes uncorrectable. The need for caution and strict control of product purity and sterility cannot be overemphasized.

There are other limitations. Suspensions are not injected directly into the bloodstream since insoluble particles can block capillaries. When the injection is into the spinal fluid or the eye or body cavities, the highest purity standards must be maintained because of the sensitivity of nerve tissue to irritant and toxic substances. It should be mentioned, incidentally, that injections are used as well for local action, in which case they are traditionally introduced subcutaneously. An example would be use of a local anesthetic. Developing technology permits maintaining localization even with injection into muscles. In one approach the drug is encapsulated in small particles of polymer that erode slowly over time for controlled release with minimal systemic effect.

The Gastrointestinal Route

Dispersion must be at the molecular level for a drug to be absorbed in the gastrointestinal system. Hence the most rapid bioavailability is from solutions, with suspensions being next and tablets and hard capsules being the slowest forms. A tablet must first disintegrate into a powder and then dissolve in the fluids in the gastrointestinal system. If the rate of dissolution is rapid, then the rate of disintegration determines how fast the drug is absorbed. If, however, the rate of dissolution is relatively slow, then the rate of disintegration may not be critical. For example, *in vivo* test results revealed that an analgesic, promoted for its rapid rate of disintegration, exhibited essentially the same rate of buildup in the bloodstream as competitive products [3].

There are disadvantages for oral dosage forms already in, or readily converted to, a state of molecular dispersion. For one thing, drugs often have a bad taste. In liquids this can be disguised using syrups and flavorings. Alternatively, soft capsules can be used which dissolve rapidly in the stomach and are essentially equivalent in rate of bioavailability to solution [4]. For tablets, coatings are used both as a barrier in the mouth and to generate a slippery surface to facilitate swallowing. Such coatings, usually sugar-based, have been perfected to achieve a pleasing appearance as well. Delayed dissolution is also needed to extend bioavailability or where the medication irritates the stomach. Here again, coated or layered tablets are designed to provide a tailored bioavailability.

The Transdermal Route

A variety of dosage forms are intended for application to the surface of the skin where the drug is absorbed and passes through the outer layers, ultimately reaching the bloodstream. Transdermal (through the skin) products are becoming increasingly popular, with patches currently available to administer scopolamine (to treat motion sickness), nitroglycerin (for angina pectoris), estradiol (a hormone to relieve menstrual symptoms), clonidine (for high blood pressure) and fentanyl (a narcotic for pain).

The rate of passage of the drug into the circulatory system is controlled by the rate of absorption and diffusion through the stratum corneum via a tortuous route of intercellular channels. Once through the stratum corneum the drug passes into the epidermis and the blood circulation of the skin (Figure 2.3). The rate of permeation depends on the level of skin hydration and the patient's age and temperature. The rate of permeation can be increased by penetration enhancers. In addition to increasing permeability of the skin, some enhancers also increase the thermodynamic activity of the penetrant. The most effective solvent for increasing skin permeability is water, but others include dimethyl sulfoxide and its analogs and laurocapram. Surfactants

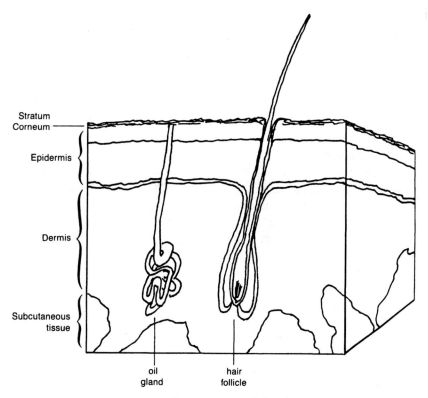

Stratum
Corneum

Epidermis

Dermis

Subcutaneous
tissue

oil
gland

hair
follicle

FIGURE 2.3. Cross section of the skin.

are also effective enhancers but they tend to cause irritation with long usage and are therefore limited in their application. A recent development is iontophoresis, a process for forcing ionized drugs through the skin by direct electric current.

The Inhalation and Nasal Routes

The administration of drugs intended to have a systemic effect by inhalation of vapors, and liquid and solid mists is well established. Examples are penicillin and other antibiotics; epinephrine, isoproterenol and similar antiasthmatic medications; and ethyl and octyl nitrate. The respiratory system allows absorption and permeation of drugs into the circulatory system at a rate that approaches intravenous injection in rapid bioavailability. Therefore, inhalation can be considered as an alternate route for virtually any drug that is given parenterally.

A critical requirement for effective systemic access by inhalation is that the particle size of a mist must initially be in the range of 1 to 5 microns to insure that even with some agglomeration, particles are small enough to be carried to the site of action in the respiratory system. The drug must also have some solubility in the fluids associated with lung tissue. Thus epinephrine bitartrate is preferred over the hydrochloride or sulfate derivative because of its higher solubility.

Nasal solutions, when dropped or sprayed into the nose, coat the nasal cavity where they can be absorbed for systemic effects. Examples of such administration include lypressin solution for the treatment of diabetes, oxytocin solution for the treatment of milk letdown prior to breast feeding, antibiotics, antihistamines, and drugs to treat asthma prophylaxis. Also being investigated for this administration route are peptides and proteins which are currently limited to injection since inactivation occurs in the gastrointestinal tract. Solutions for nasal administration are formulated to match as closely as possible the chemistry of nasal secretions to encourage normal ciliary activity. Important factors are isotonicity (similar colligative or osmotic properties) and a pH in the range of 5.5 to 6.5.

The Rectal Route

Absorption of drugs in the rectum is similar to that in other body cavities. The drug must first dissolve in the rectal fluids and then permeate the rectal mucosa. Since the drug will partition itself between the vehicle used for insertion in the rectum and the rectal fluids, such vehicle-drug combinations must be carefully chosen to achieve optimum bioavailability. Studies made on aspirin and aspirin derivatives suggest about equal bioavailability for oral and rectal administration. However, broadly based equivalency has not been established, and rectal absorption is thought to be more erratic.

Permeation through the rectal mucosa is the rate-determining step for drugs which dissolve rapidly. A number of substances will effectively enhance permeation. Some, such as bile salts and anti-inflammatories, increase water influx and efflux rates across the mucosa. Surfactants increase surface wetting and improve membrane permeability. Circulatory system access is different for different locations in the rectum. Veins that are present in the lower and middle portions bypass the liver so that drugs absorbed in these areas pass directly into the vena cava.

Examples of drugs administered rectally for systemic effects are sedatives, tranquilizers and analgesics.

Packaging Needs

All the routes used for systemic access have demanding requirements which often can only be fulfilled by complex and precisely structured and formulated drug products. For such precision products, preservation of the original pristine state of the product is a critical packaging need. Other generalizations are not possible since the different administration routes are served by quite different dosage forms, all of which, along with their packaging needs, are covered in the next section.

DOSAGE FORMS

The description of dosage forms that follow is grouped by physical state since this determines primarily the packages that are used. Within each physical state, dosage forms are further grouped according to the mode or site of administration. The descriptive material includes the methods of preparation of the physical state, descriptions of each dosage form within that state and the packaging needs for the physical state.

SOLIDS

Solids include finely divided powders, microencapsulated powders and loosely agglomerated powders or granules, tablets and caplets, hard and soft capsules, and suppositories.

Powders, Microencapsulated
Powders, and Granules

Preparation

Powders

Powder preparation involves two processes—the isolation of coarse, aggregated substances and the reduction of particle size.

Isolation of the coarse substance is generally from a solution by precipitation or spray drying. A number of approaches are used for particle size reduction since the physical nature of the coarse substance varies. Some drug substances are heat sensitive or have low melting points and cannot be processed in ways, such as milling, that generate heat. Others are fibrous in nature and resist breakdown by pressure or impact methods. Some substances are very hard and cause severe abrasion of grinding surfaces.

Usually, size reduction is accomplished in several, successive operations (see Figure 2.4):

1. Coarse crushing is done with roller and impact crushers.
2. Intermediate grinding is performed using cutter blades rotating through fixed discs, rotating hammers or rollers.
3. Fine grinding is done using rollers, cutters, hammers, grinding stones or plates, balls tumbled in a rotating container, fluid energy mills where particles are subjected to high velocity gas streams or centrifugal pulverizers where particles are flung against impact surfaces. Grinding mills are often coupled with screens that separate out the larger particles for recycling through the mill.
4. For creating mixtures of powders, various dry blending techniques are used including rotating drums containing baffles, double cones or twin shells joined as a V and rotated about an axis cutting across the arms of the V, fixed vessels with ribbon or paddle stirrers and containers where powders are fluidized and mixed by air.

Microencapsulated Powders

Microencapsulation, the coating of very small solid particles or liquid droplets, is done in a variety of ways. In one of the simplest, the particles or droplets are dispersed in a solution of a coating material under conditions where the coating material deposits out by phase separation onto the core particle or droplet. The resultant product can be recovered as a free flowing powder after isolation and hardening of the coating by drying or chemical cross linking. In another approach, particles are spray coated and dried while suspended and agitated in a fluidized bed.

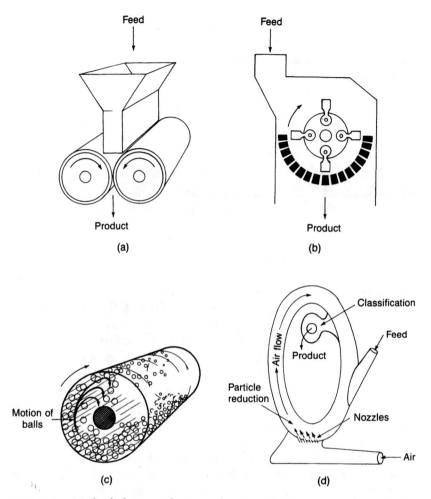

FIGURE 2.4. Methods for particle size reduction. (a) Horizontal roller mill; (b) swing hammer crusher (cross section); (c) ball mill; (d) fluid energy mill.

Granules

Granules are prepared from a moist, agglomerated mass which is subdivided by passage through a screen and then dried. Effervescent granules and powders are formulated with sodium bicarbonate and a mild acid (citric or tartaric) or sodium biphosphate along with the active ingredients. The duration of contact of these formulations with water during preparation must be limited to leave sufficient unreacted ingredients to produce effervescence when mixed with water for administration. The right amount of water for granulation is achieved by heating the powder and driving off the water of hydration from the citric acid. Alternatively, a small amount of water is added to produce a workable mass which is then dried and ground to produce a powder or granule. A more sophisticated approach is to suspend the powders in a fluidized bed to which water is added to achieve the right level of agglomeration with minimum effervescent reaction. This eliminates separate drying and grinding steps, provides better control, and allows continuous processing.

Oral Powders and Granules

Grinding natural materials into powders was one of the first methods of preparing crude drugs. While traditional medicines are still prepared and dispensed this way in many cultures (such as the Chinese), capsules and tablets are the preferred dosage form for the more potent synthetic drugs. Powders are difficult to handle; many are hydroscopic or deliquescent. Accurate administration from multiple unit packages is difficult. Most drugs have an unpleasant taste. Nevertheless, powdered dosage forms persist because they permit flexibility in compounding and because the powder can be mixed with water just prior to administration. When mixed with water, effervescent granules and powders release carbon dioxide, which helps to mask the taste of the active ingredients. Furthermore, powders such as laxatives and antacids can be added to soft foods.

Topical Powders

These preparations, also called dusting powders, are intended for local action when applied to various parts of the body as lubricants, protectives, absorbents, antiseptics, antipruritics, and astringents. Care must be taken to minimize factors that could cause irritation, especially of traumatized areas. Topical powders are usually passed through a 100 mesh screen to eliminate grit.

Sterile Powders for Injection

Some pharmaceuticals for injection are supplied as powders because of instability in solution. These are dissolved in water just prior to use. For drugs, such as some biologicals, that will not tolerate the isolation and drying conditions used for normal powder preparation, the powder is produced by freeze-drying (lyophilization). In this process a solvent is evaporated by means of a vacuum applied at ambient or lower temperatures. Often this process takes place in the final packaging container.

Tablets

Tablets are made in a variety of shapes (e.g., round, spherical, oval, oblong) and edge configurations as shown in Figure 2.5. *Caplet* is a name given to the oblong shape which resembles a capsule. Sizes and weights vary depending on the amount of drug in the dose and the mode of administration. They are prepared by compression or molding.

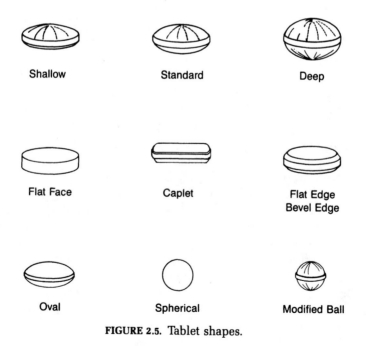

Shallow   Standard   Deep

Flat Face   Caplet   Flat Edge
Bevel Edge

Oval   Spherical   Modified Ball

FIGURE 2.5. Tablet shapes.

Preparation

Compressed Tablets

Compressed tablets are made by compaction of powdered or granular substances. Additives are employed to facilitate cohesion and lubrication in the making of the tablet and later disintegration in use. Additives also dilute and add color. The manufacturing process consists of two basic steps—mixing of ingredients, and compaction into a tablet. In the most widely used mixing method—wet granulation—the active drug and additives are first dry blended in large scale blenders such as twin-shell rotary blenders, stirred vessels, and fluidized beds. A water solution of the tablet binder is then added to produce a wet agglomerate of the right consistency for processing into tablets. Where justified by a high production volume, screw extruders are used for continuous blending and wet mixing. The wet mass is next screened or milled to improve particle size uniformity and dried in ovens or fluidized beds using warm air.

Some steps in this process can be eliminated by spraying a solution of the formulation ingredients into a fluidized bed containing suspended inert particles or the active drug (to build up granules) and then drying, all in one piece of equipment.

In both the wet granulation and fluidized bed processes, residual granule moisture is controlled to a level that maintains binders in an optimum state while minimizing static electricity buildup, but a level that is not deleterious to moisture sensitive drugs. A final screening to remove large particles is followed by the addition of a lubricant, such as talc, which promotes easy flow into the tablet forming equipment and prevents adhesion of the formulation to machine parts. Where the active drug or other formulation ingredients have inherent binding capability, and particularly for moisture sensitive drugs, a dry granulation process can be used. Here, air must first be removed from the dry mixture by compressing it into 1-inch cylinders or by compaction in roller mills. Then the compacted material is disintegrated into granules. Processing of the granules proceeds as for the wet granulation process. Aspirin and some antacid preparations can be prepared this way. Finally, direct compression of a powdered drug formulation is sometimes possible when the mixture has the characteristics necessary for good tablet formation.

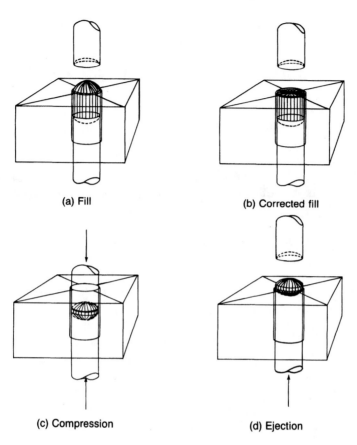

(a) Fill   (b) Corrected fill

(c) Compression   (d) Ejection

FIGURE 2.6. Tablet making by compression.

The basic machine for tablet formation is shown in Figure 2.6 and consists of a cavity (cylindrical in shape for round tablets), open at both ends, into which two opposing punches are driven under pressure to compact the formulation. The shape of the punch faces and the die cavity determines the shape of the tablet. Raised patterns on the punch face produce scoring and/or monograms. In operation, the cavity with the lower punch inserted is filled with granules using a mechanism that delivers a measured quantity and also scrapes off the excess. The upper punch is then driven downward with sufficient pressure to achieve optimum compaction.

Finally, the upper punch is withdrawn and the lower punch is driven upward, ejecting the finished tablet from the die cavity.

Any remaining fine powder or excess granules are removed by screening and vacuuming the tablets. This basic operation can be extended from single to multiple sets of punches and dies in rotary machines with automatically controlled cycles for filling and activating compaction and ejection. High-speed tablet machines can produce as many as 14,000 tablets per minute depending on granulation formulation.

Multilayered tablets are produced by adding separate granulations to the tablet cavity in steps with intervening compaction followed by a final compression stroke. Alternatively, a precompressed tablet is placed in a second machine which adds another layer.

Molded Tablets

Molded tablets or tablet triturates are prepared to achieve rapid dissolution in water. Tablet triturates are made by filling cylindrical cavities in a plate with the wetted formulation and ejecting the formed tablets by means of a second plate with pegs that match the positions of the cavities as shown in Figure 2.7. This process is either operated by hand with up to 500 cavities per plate or is automated using machines that perform the sequential steps by indexing cavities to appropriate stations for filling, smoothing the top surface and ejecting the finished tablet. Production rates for such machines can be up to 2500 tablets per minute.

Tablet Coating

The most popular coating process employs a perforated drum rotating on its horizontal axis to provide a tumbling movement of the tablets. Coating solutions are normally sprayed onto the tablets. Drying air is introduced through the perforations in the drum and exhausted from the inner space above the tablets, or is introduced from above the tablet bed and exhausted through the drum perforations (Figure 2.8a). Tablets tend to move quickly through the spray application zone, receiving a layer of coating over a portion of the tablet surface which in turn is partially transferred to neighboring tablets before drying begins. Repeated application-transfer-drying cycles build up the coating thickness

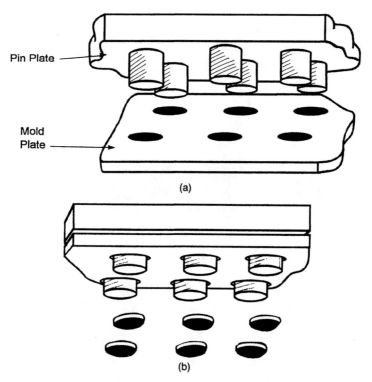

Pin Plate

Mold
Plate

(a)

(b)

FIGURE 2.7. Molding tablet triturates: (a) filled mold; (b) ejected triturates.

and uniformity to the desired level. The coating process is operated in both batch and continuous modes.

A number of variations on this process are used. In pan coaters, the pan is rotated about its vertical axis at a small angle to the horizontal plane. Coating solution is added both by spraying and by hand ladeling onto the tablet bed. Drying air is sometimes introduced into the interior of the bed using perforated tubes to improve drying efficiency as depicted in Figure 2.8b. Fluidized beds are also employed. Here, tablets are suspended and agitated within a cylindrical container using a column of drying air (Figure 2.9). Typically the movement of the tablets is upward at the core of the cylinder, then outward toward the wall at the top of the bed and finally down in a cascade to return to the bottom of the column. Coating solution is sprayed either from the bottom onto the rising tablets or from the top onto the cascading tablets.

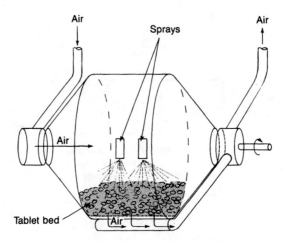

FIGURE 2.8a. Drum coater for tablets.

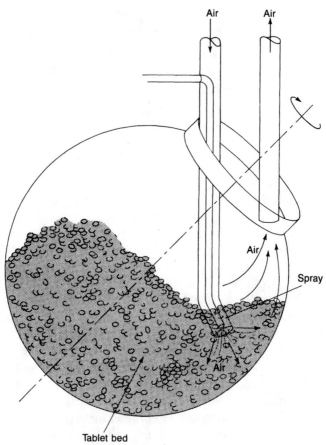

FIGURE 2.8b. Pan coater with immersion tube.

42

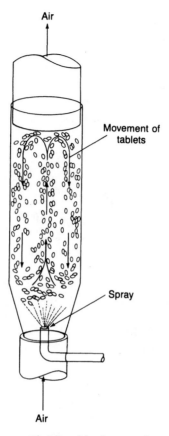

Air

Movement of
tablets

Spray

Air

FIGURE 2.9. Fluidized bed coater for tablets.

Sugar coating is widely used and normally consists of multiple coating steps to achieve all of the desired coating properties. A seal coating of such substances as shellac or protein is first applied to prevent penetration of water from the subsequent sugar syrups into the tablet which can cause softening and possibly deterioration of the drug. Next a subcoating of sugar solution and thickeners is repeatedly applied with intermittent applications of insoluble powders such as talc, kaolin or starch to round edges and build up tablet size. Then a series of smoothing and coloring coats, also based on syrup, is applied. Typically, the last coatings in this phase are clear. The final coating consists of waxes applied as powders or solutions to provide luster to the tablet.

Film coatings are applied in much the same way as sugar-coatings with the principal difference being the formulation ingredients. For film coatings various polymeric substances are used to form continuous films. Some formulations are applied from organic solvent systems while others are water soluble. The properties of the coating film can be modified by the addition of plasticizers and adhesion promoters as well as the usual additives to achieve opaqueness and color.

Oral Tablets

Tablets make up 75% of all solid dosage forms, hard capsules comprise 23% of the total, and soft capsules 2%. Advantages of tablets for the consumer are accuracy of dosage, convenience, relatively pleasant administration, and ready portability. For the manufacturer the advanced tablet technologies permit economic preparation, combination of many attributes by designed layering and coating and convenient handling, packaging and shipping.

The formulations for compressed tablets have been developed to maximize ease of disintegration in the gastrointestinal system. Disintegration can be further enhanced by the addition of a deep slot in the tablet during the compaction cycle. Layered tablets permit alteration of bioavailability and protection of a sensitive core drug. Layers also allow the separation of different drugs or of different formulations of the same drug so that a single dose provides sequential drug release in different parts of the gastrointestinal tract. Layered separation is also used for incompatible drug mixtures.

In general, coatings for compressed tablets provide an attractive finish for the tablet with the addition of color, a glossy uniform surface and printing. Coatings are also used as an alternative to layering where incompatibility is a problem or sequential release is desired. Sugar coatings cover up objectionable tastes, odors or appearances, create a slipperiness in the mouth that eases swallowing, and protect the formulation from oxygen. Water soluble film coatings provide advantages similar to sugar coatings. Polymers used for such coatings include hydroxypropyl methylcellulose, methyl hydroxyethylcellulose, povidone, polyethylene glycols, and acrylate polymers. Enteric coatings provide delayed bioavailability to protect the stomach from irritating drugs. Typical film forming substances used for enteric coatings are cellulose acetate phthalate, acrylic resins, and phthalate derivatives of polyvinyl acetate.

For sublingual administration, both molded and compressed tablet preparations are formulated to dissolve rapidly in the mouth as is required for drugs such as nitroglycerin, isoproterenol hydrochloride (a relaxant for heart and smooth muscles), and erythrityl tetranitrate (for treatment of chronic angina). Water soluble drug vehicles including lactose and dextrose are employed, and the tablet is generally softer than compressed tablets.

Other Tablets

Effervescent tablets, like effervescent powders, contain sodium bicarbonate and organic acids such as tartaric or citric. Upon contact with water, carbon dioxide is produced, providing effervescence and facilitating disintegration. The ingredients are essentially all soluble and create a liquid dosage form when mixed with water.

Vaginal suppositories containing drugs such as metronidazole (used to treat anaerobic bacterial infections) are sometimes prepared as compressed tablets. The diluent used is usually lactose. Buccal tablets are small, flat, and oval shaped and are inserted in the buccal cavity where the slow dissolution desired is attained by means of hard compression of the tablet. Dispensing tablets of potent drugs can be supplied in tablet form as a convenient way to extemporaneously prepare powders or liquids.

Capsules

A capsule is a hard or soft, water soluble shell that contains either a powder or liquid. A hard capsule is made as two halves, filled in a separate operation and closed by slipping one half over the other. A soft capsule, by contrast, is formed, filled and sealed in a continuous, single operation that generally encapsulates a liquid product.

Hard Capsules

Preparation

The dominant material used in the manufacture of hard capsules is gelatin derived from acid processing of pork skins or from alkaline processing of animal bones and skins. By blending these two varieties, optimum solution viscosity and shell strength are achieved. Additives include colorants and sometimes opacifiers. As shown in Figure 2.10, capsule shells are produced by dipping a pin into a gelatin solution and drying the coating under precisely controlled temperature and humidity. Solution viscosity, dipping conditions, and residual moisture content determine wall thickness, which must be precisely controlled to insure a proper fit of the two halves of the capsule. The level of residual moisture content is also critical for the physical properties of the capsule: at a low level capsules are brittle, and at the high end they are flaccid and lose shape. The formed, dried shell is stripped from the pin, trimmed to the proper length and fitted into the second half for storage and shipment. In a completely

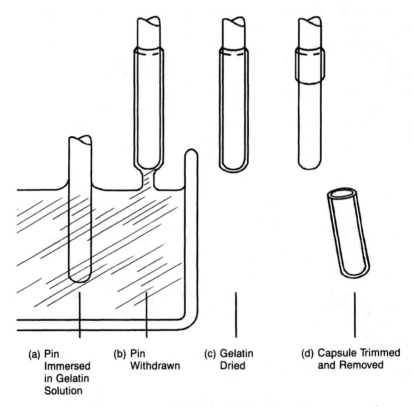

| (a) Pin Immersed in Gelatin Solution | (b) Pin Withdrawn | (c) Gelatin Dried | (d) Capsule Trimmed and Removed |

FIGURE 2.10. The making of hard capsules.

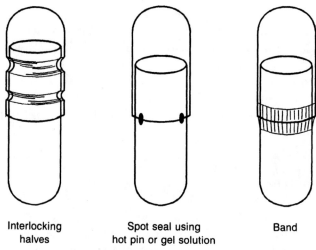

| Interlocking halves | Spot seal using hot pin or gel solution | Band |

FIGURE 2.11. Sealing methods for hard capsules.

automatic commercial operation, typically 150 pairs of rotating pins are dipped and then dried, first in cool air and then in ovens. The shell halves are then trimmed, joined and ejected from the machine. A full cycle requires 45 minutes. An alternative, recently developed process for making hard capsule shells is injection molding of extrudable starch formulations. More precise control of capsule dimensions and higher productivity are advantages of this process.

Capsules are made in a range of standard sizes with capacities of from 30–600 mg of powdered product. Filling on a semiautomatic basis is accomplished by machines that have outputs as high as 160,000 capsules per hour. The first step in the operation is to place the body halves of the capsules into holes in a ring. Each body half is then indexed around to fit under a filling unit that delivers the drug product and scrapes off the excess. A matching plate with cap halves in place is then brought into position so that the two halves are joined and pressed together. Filled capsules are cleaned by mild agitation in the presence of sodium chloride and by rolling on a cloth surface. Powder formulations generally contain a diluent (e.g., lactose or calcium carbonate) to match drug concentration to capsule filling volume, and a lubricant (e.g., stearates) to facilitate powder flow and capsule filling.

Several techniques can be used to insure that filled, closed capsules do not come apart during handling (Figure 2.11). In one approach, the ends of the capsule halves are shaped to form inter-locking, matched rings that snap together when the halves are joined. Capsule halves can also be sealed together either by weld-ing through the use of a hot pin placed against the capsule joint, by gelatin solution, or a gelatin band. One of these sealing tech-niques is now mandatory to achieve tamper evidence. Also, band-ing has been shown to greatly improve the barrier of the capsule to oxygen penetration [5].

Oral Hard Capsules

Hard capsules are tasteless, convenient, easy to administer, easy to swallow, and even chewable. In general, capsules dissolve more readily in the stomach than tablets since they usually contain un-compacted powders. Both solids and liquids can be placed in cap-sules, but solids (usually powders but may include granules, pellets and tablets) predominate. For extemporaneous filling, cap-sules allow tailoring of the dose to individual patient needs. There are some limitations with capsules: efflorescent materials can soften them to an undesirable degree and deliquescent powders can cause embrittlement.

Powder formulation requirements are relatively simple com-pared to compressed tablets so that capsules are often used for new drugs during clinical trials. Additives are used, however, to facilitate filling at high speeds, which in many cases requires a free flowing powder that readily slips past machine surfaces. Thus, cornstarch is added to acetylsalicylic acid to enhance flow-ability while stearates are used to provide lubrication. On the other hand, some filling machines form and insert a pellet into the capsule. In this case, additives such as microcrystalline cellu-lose that aid compaction and mineral oil to increase cohesion are used. These additives can affect bioavailability but not as strongly as in tablets.

Various process modifications can be used to add properties to the basic capsule. Enteric coatings are used to delay dissolution. Separation of incompatible substances is accomplished in cap-sules by encasing one substance in a small hard or soft capsule or tablet. This is first placed in the capsule, which is then filled with the second substance in powder form. Recent machine develop-ments permit filling with liquids and semisolids. Generally the drug formulation is either a semisolid at room temperature which is melted for filling or is converted to liquid by the shearing forces of pumping. In either case, it is necessary for the liquid to solidify sufficiently after filling to prevent leakage. Sealing of the capsule with a gelatin band is also effective in retaining a liquid fill.

Soft Capsules

Soft capsules consist of two matching halves of a sphere or ellipsoid hermetically sealed to encase a drug which is usually a liquid but can be a paste, tablet or pellet. The shell is made of gelatin plasticized with 30–40% glycerin or sorbitol to enhance formability and water solubility.

Preparation

The process for manufacturing soft capsules consists of forming two layers of warm gelatin film into the capsule shape by injecting the drug product under pressure between the layers and thermoforming the films into two matching mold cavities on either side of the film sandwich. The edges of the shaped capsule are sealed and the finished capsule is cut out of the film layers as pressure forces the mold rims together. Continuous manufacture is accomplished by feeding two films into the nip of two rotating wheels that bring together matching die faces to form the capsule mold as shown in Figure 2.12. Precise synchronization allows product to be injected at the film nip point as the edges of the capsule are being sealed up to the injection port; complete sealing and edge cutting occurs as the films advance through the nip. At the exit of the nip, capsules drop onto a collection screen and residual film is captured for reuse.

While premanufactured gelatin films can be used to feed the continuous process, usually the films are cast from a fluid mass just upstream of the capsule formation step. To form this mass, the gelatin is further plasticized with an excess of water and maintained at about 60°C. Other ingredients in the formulation may include preservatives, colorants, opacifiers, and flavorings. Film forms as the gelatin mass flows by gravity through a slot and solidifies on a drum. When the gelatin film is lubricated with min-

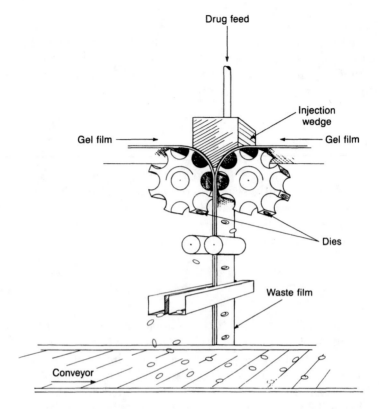

FIGURE 2.12. Continuous process for making soft capsules.

eral oil to facilitate easy movement over machine surfaces, the oil must be removed using a naptha wash of the capsules just after manufacture. This step is followed by drying to a residual moisture content of 6 to 10%, the equilibrium level for an RH of 20 to 30%. The final step is heat branding or printing of the capsule.

Typically, the drug product intended for encasement in soft capsules is dissolved or suspended in a liquid, but there are limitations. Liquids such as water or alcohols that are water miscible and volatile cannot be used since they can readily permeate the capsule walls. Gelatin plasticizers such as glycerin or glycols cannot be major constituents of the drug formulation since these would increase the susceptibility of the capsule to the effects of heat and humidity.

Oral Soft Capsules

The advantages of oral soft capsules are easy portability and accurately controlled administration of liquid medications. In addition, they act more quickly than hard capsules or tablets because the hermetic seal is rapidly broken down by gastric fluids and because liquids are more rapidly absorbed than solids. Enhanced bioavailability for soft capsules versus tablets is cited for chlormethiazole [6], digoxin (for treatment of heart failure) [7,8], papaverine (for vascodilation) [9], and diazepam (for the treatment of anxiety disorders) [10]. Similar studies generally showed bioavailability for soft capsules equivalent to unencapsulated liquids and superior to hard capsules. For oral applications, capsule shells are plasticized at the lower end of the range (30–35%) to achieve the right balance of hardness and solubility. Coatings based on cellulosic derivatives have been developed for soft capsules to delay bioavailability.

The effect of the gelatin shell on the encased drug can be both positive and negative. Gelatin is an excellent oxygen barrier and can be opacified to eliminate light. Vitamins exhibit enhanced stability in soft capsules versus tablets. However, some interaction of the drug and the gelatin is possible. The usual problem is the absorption of moisture from the shell which can lead to chemical changes in the drug and embrittlement of the shell. In some cases the form of the drug can be selected to minimize this effect (such as using procaine penicillin instead of potassium penicillin), or the drug formulation can be modified (for example by changing the pH of the solution). Another approach to reduce interaction is microencapsulation.

Nonoral Soft Capsules

Soft capsules are also used as suppositories for rectal and vaginal administration of drugs. Rectal administration is especially useful for pediatric and geriatric patients and for drugs that irritate the gastrointestinal system. Again, the major advantage of the soft capsule over other dosage forms is rapid bioavailability. For example, in one study, the concentration of the analgesic, acetaminophen, in the urine four hours after administration was 5 to 8 times greater for the soft capsule than for a traditional suppository [6].

In tube form, soft capsules serve as a convenient, specialty, single dose package for ointments intended for topical, ophthalmic, otic, and rectal administration. Long acting nitroglycerin ointments applied transdermally are an example of this application. For all of these applications, capsule shells contain higher levels of plasticizer (35–40%) to maximize softness and solubility.

Suppositories

While tablets and capsules are sometimes used as suppositories, this dosage form is normally a molded shape specifically designed for insertion into body orifices (the rectum, vagina, and urethra) where the solid melts, softens or dissolves at body temperature.

Preparation

Typically, oils that are solids at room temperature are used as the base to contain the therapeutic additives and to facilitate administration. The choice of the base substance depends on the site of insertion and on the properties of the therapeutic additives. While cocoa butter is a common choice for rectal administration since it melts readily and is nonirritating, it leaves a residue and is not appropriate for vaginal use. Here, water soluble bases such as polyglycols and glycerinated gels are used. These water soluble bases are not often used in rectal suppositories because the rate of dissolution and drug release is too slow. Cocoa butter is not miscible with body fluids. Thus, dissolution of fat-soluble drugs intended for systemic action is inhibited. Alternatives to cocoa butter include a variety of modified vegetable oils.

One method of preparing suppositories is to incorporate the finely divided added substances into the base, work the solid mixture at room temperature and then shape the mass. Shaping can either be by hand rolling or compression molding. In the latter approach, the mass is forced by pressure into a mold opening followed by opening of the mold and removal. In large scale operations, the mass is screw fed into a cavity from which it is forced by a hydraulically operated piston into the mold. Another method is compounding the mixture as a liquid at elevated temperature followed by solidification on cooling in a mold. Rectal suppositories are generally tapered at one or both ends whereas vaginal suppositories are usually globular or oviform.

Rectal Suppositories

The largest use is probably for hemorrhoid treatment by local actions of the cocoa butter (as a protectant and palliative) and of medicinal additives. Suppositories are also broadly used to administer drugs intended for systemic action. Rectal administration is particularly advantageous for the very young, the very old, or other patients for whom oral administration is difficult. Drugs incorporated in rectal suppositories include sedatives, tranquilizers, and analgesics. Other specific applications are the use of pentobarbital sodium and pyrilamine maleate for the treatment of nausea and vomiting, and the use of various mixtures such as caffeine and ergotamine for the treatment of migraine headaches [11,12].

Nonrectal Suppositories

Vaginal and uterine suppositories are used for both local and systemic effects. Extensive drug absorption has been shown to occur in the vagina. Progesterone preparations are extemporaneously compounded into vaginal suppositories and are also available commercially for intrauterine administration.

Packaging Needs for
Solid Dosage Forms

The most significant characteristic of finely divided powders from the packaging viewpoint is the very high surface area-to-volume ratio. This means that moisture or oxygen pickup will be very rapid as compared to more agglomerated forms. Thus, protection from moisture is the principal packaging need for oral powders since many are hydroscopic leading to agglomeration and even solidification. Effervescent powders and granules react with moisture. Granules tend to be very fragile and easily broken down into undesirable fines during handling and shipping. Also, particles tend to have sharp corners which can puncture and erode the surface of packaging materials. For powders intended for injection or ophthalmic applications, all of the requirements described earlier for sterile pharmaceuticals apply.

Tablets are often fragile or complex in structure to achieve ready disintegration and/or controlled rates of absorption. Protection from physical damage or breakdown during handling and shipping is critical. Uncoated tablets are more fragile than coated tablets but coatings can be abraded or chipped, which alters the desired pattern of systemic administration. Protection of tablets from moisture is often necessary. For some, moisture dramatically changes the rate of disintegration by altering the physical structure of the tablet. In laboratory studies, subsequent drying did not always return the solid to its original state. Also, moisture can deteriorate a coating, causing it to discolor or become mottled and dulled.

Hard capsules are not particularly fragile or sensitive to moisture. The moisture content of soft capsules, on the other hand, must be maintained within a reasonable range to avoid embrittlement at the low end or softening and sticking at the upper end. The absorption of moisture is a particular problem in tropical environments as is fungal attack. Protection from both is important.

Suppositories intended to melt readily must be protected from heat and are usually stored at controlled room temperature. Those that dissolve rather than melt generally melt well above room temperature, but they are moisture sensitive.

LIQUIDS

This section includes pure liquids, solutions, suspensions, and emulsions except those administered as aerosols.

Preparation

Pure Liquids

Few pure liquids are used as dosage forms. Preparation generally involves purification by processes such as distillation and filtration. While not considered a medicinal liquid, water is a common vehicle or solvent in most liquid dosage forms and the

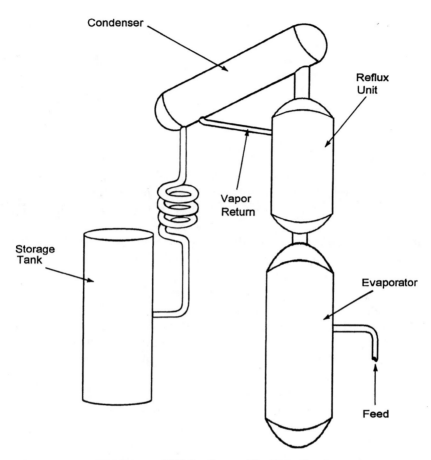

FIGURE 2.13. Still for the purification of water.

preparation of pharmaceutical grade (purified water) is illustrative of the practices that are employed for other liquids.

The main impurities in water are salts of calcium, iron, magnesium, manganese and sodium, silica, organics, and microorganisms. A still for the distillation of water (Figure 2.13) consists of (1) an evaporator where heat is applied to bring the fluid to a boiling point and to achieve a high rate of evaporation; (2) a head space above the boiler where vapor condenses and refluxes, allowing nonvolatile material to return to the boiler; (3) a means for eliminating volatile impurities in the vapor; and (4) a condenser where the vapor is liquified by the removal of heat. This process will produce pure, sterile water provided it is controlled properly and provided the equipment is sterile at the outset. Proper storage is critical to retain sterility.

Alternatively, impurities may be removed from water by passing it through ion-exchange columns containing either cationic or anionic exchange resins. However, phosphates and organic debris in exchange columns are excellent growth media for microorganisms, and care must be taken to destroy bacteria in the column prior to use.

Reverse osmosis is another purification process that may be used. Pure solvent, separated from a solution by a membrane permeable only to the solvent, will tend to flow through the semipermeable membrane into the solution. If pressure is applied to the solution that is equal to the osmotic pressure, flow will cease. If the pressure is greater than the osmotic pressure, flow is reversed and pure solvent (purified water) flows from the solution (impure water) to the pure solvent side of the membrane. Pore size in semipermeable membranes is generally small enough to eliminate larger organic molecules and microorganisms larger than about 100 Å in diameter. However, larger openings can develop and microorganisms can quickly multiply within the process. Often combinations of these various purification approaches are used.

While these procedures will produce *purified water*, the design of the still and operating procedures are more stringent for purer versions such as *water for injection*. For the latter, important process elements include low vapor velocity in the boiler, efficient separation of the condensing vapor and the distilling liquid, continuous removal of volatile impurities, and appropriately lined vessels and other parts. Also, water for injection is usually not stored but used directly from the purifying process. USP monographs contain requirements for *water for injection* and *sterile water for injection* that are intended for packaged sterilized products. Such requirements include maximum solids and ionic contaminant levels.

Solutions

A solution consists of a solvent, almost always water for pharmaceutical preparations, in which volatile, liquid, or solid substances (solutes) are dissolved, that is, completely dispersed at the molecular or ionic level. Dissolution is achieved by addition of the solute to the solvent with agitation sufficient to attain molecular dispersion. For difficult-to-dissolve substances which can tolerate heat, the temperature of the solvent can be elevated. Where a saturated solution is desired, an excess of solute is added or the solvent is heated and then cooled, allowing the excess to precipitate out. In either case the excess material must be removed by filtration from the final preparation or the clear liquid decanted off if the excess material forms a distinct second phase. Sometimes solutions are produced by reacting two or more solutes in the solvent. An example is aluminum subacetate, used for topical applications, where aluminum sulfate is mixed with calcium carbonate and acetic acid.

Aromatic waters are saturated solutions of volatile organic substances or other aromatic substances which are prepared by distilling a mixture of purified water and the added substance, allowing the distillate to carry the aromatic oil or by shaking water with the oil. To improve efficiency of dispersion, oils are first mixed with fine powders such as talc to increase surface area and that mixture is shaken with water. Examples of aromatic substances used are peppermint, anise, cinnamon, dill, caraway and fennel. When alcohol is used to extract crude drugs from vegetable, animal or inorganic matter, the resulting solutions are called tinctures (e.g., tincture of iodine and benzoin tincture).

Syrups are sweet, viscous solutions, generally of sugars, polyols or polysaccharides, in water. Sometimes alcohol is added both as a preservative and as an aid in dissolving medicinal solutes. Generally, the concentration of sugar is close to but below the saturation level. A high sugar concentration retards the growth of microorganisms but too high a level can lead to crystallization of part of the sucrose as temperature decreases. Syrups are prepared in glass-lined tanks with mechanical agitators by either heating all the ingredients in water or, when drug substances are heat sensitive, adding substances to the previously prepared syrup. Care must be taken to avoid overheating syrups since sucrose is readily converted by heat to its optical isomer, levulose, which is darker in color and has a greater tendency to ferment. Sterilization of syrups in an autoclave generally leads to some caramelization. Preservatives are used to inhibit growth of mold and bacteria especially for low concentrations of sugar in the syrup.

After their preparation, all solutions must be filtered to remove foreign matter and excess solute. Filtration can also be effective for the reduction of microorganisms.

Emulsions

An emulsion is a liquid consisting of one discontinuous phase dispersed as small droplets in a second continuous phase. Such a dispersion is generally unstable so that a third component, an emulsifying agent, is added. The most common pharmaceutical emulsions are oil dispersed in water using thickeners (e.g., cellulose derivatives and polyglycols) and surfactants (e.g., sodium lauryl sulfate). Drugs can be dissolved in either the oil or the water phase. Since growth of microorganisms is favored in the aqueous phase of an emulsion, water soluble preservatives are usually added; however, pairs of preservatives are often used since microorganisms can also grow in the oil phase. The normal technique is to dissolve the various additives in the phase in which they are soluble prior to mixing.

Mechanical energy is required to achieve a satisfactory emulsion containing small droplets of the discontinuous phase. The higher the energy input, the lower the amount of emulsifying agent required for stability. A wide variety of devices are used to achieve dispersion. Agitated vessels employ propellers or paddles with high powered drive shafts and often utilize baffles attached to the vessel walls to increase efficiency. Also used are colloid mills, shown in Figure 2.14, consisting of a high speed rotor revolving against a stator with very narrow clearances and homogenizers where high shear forces are achieved by forcing the mixture through a valve onto an impact surface.

Suspensions

When water insoluble drugs are administered in liquid form, a suspension of the finely divided solid drug in water is usually used. As with emulsions, the stability of the suspension depends on the particle size of the solid, the viscosity of the liquid and the presence of a dispersing agent, a surfactant. Fine particle sizes are achieved by techniques described earlier for powders. The suspending liquid may be thickened using cellulose derivatives.

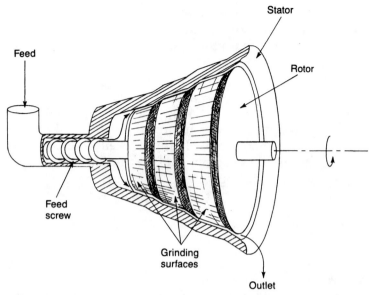

FIGURE 2.14. Colloid mill.

Oral Liquids

Oral liquids have the advantage over solids of being easier to swallow and over tablets of having more rapid bioavailability. On the other hand, administering the dose is less convenient and more prone to error. While liquids expose the mouth to the often unpleasant taste of drugs, flavored syrups can mask most of these tastes and are frequently used as a vehicle. Syrups are widely used for pediatric preparations such as those containing aspirin. OTC cough syrups contain a wide variety of ingredients which can include demulcents, expectorants and sedatives; prescription formulations can include codeine phosphate. While many oral liquids contain minor amounts of nonaqueous solvents such as alcohol, in some preparations the nonaqueous content is a significant portion of the formulation weight. Elixirs, for example, contain 20 to 25% to aid solubility.

Some drugs are either unstable or insoluble in solvents appropriate for internal administration. In such cases, suspensions are used since drugs tend to be more chemically stable in suspensions as compared to solutions. Their fine particle size makes drugs in suspension nearly as bioavailable as drugs in solution. Unpleasant tastes are considerably reduced or absent in suspensions although flavorings are often added. For children, suspensions may be frozen and given as flavored popsicles. Antibiotics are often supplied as suspensions. Some unstable drugs must be made up into solutions or suspensions extemporaneously for immediate use or for very short storage periods. Typical of this category are several antibiotics including cloxacillin sodium, nafcillin sodium, and vancomycin. Highly thickened suspensions are called magmas or milks (e.g., milk of magnesia). They tend to settle out readily on standing.

Topical Liquids

Liquids are easier to spread and more compatible with the skin than powders. Emulsion preparations with oil as the dominant phase can be applied most evenly since the thin film of sebum on the skin favors the oily phase. Liquids can also provide a soothing and protective cover for irritated skin. The rare examples of solutions used for topical applications are collodion as a protective layer (a solution of a nitrocellulose in a mixture of ethanol and ethyl ether) and some liniments. When suspensions are used topically, particle size is kept small, approaching colloidal dimensions, to enhance the soothing effect on inflamed tissue. The classic topical suspension is calamine lotion. Other lotions include antibiotics, steroids, keratolytics and scabicides as well as skin moisturizers and protectors.

Ophthalmic Liquids

Solutions are the most common vehicle for administering drugs to the eye since they feature rapid absorption of the drug, uniformity, and minimum physical interference with vision. On the other hand, retention of the liquid on the eye surface may be too brief, so thickeners such as methylcellulose are sometimes employed. Suspensions offer a longer contact time since particles are retained in the cul-de-sac. Absorption takes place only for the drug which is in solution. As dissolved drug is withdrawn, it is replaced by additional dissolution from the solid particles. Since this dissolution is generally the step that limits rate of absorption, small particle size facilitates rapid absorption. Small particle size also diminishes irritation and reduces excessive tearing, which washes out the dose.

Sterility is critical for ophthalmic liquids. Freedom of solutions from particulates is also important. The vehicle for ophthalmic liquids is ideally isotonic (equal in osmotic pressure to a 0.9% sodium chloride solution) and matches the pH of tears to avoid irritating eye tissues. Such vehicles are solutions consisting of sterile distilled water that contains either sodium chloride, boric acid or phosphates (sometimes mixed) and a preservative. The pH may have to be compromised to accommodate the stability needs of additives. Examples of drugs used in ophthalmic solutions are anesthetics (cocaine, phenacaine, procaine, tetracaine and piperocaine), smooth muscle relaxants (epinephrine, phenylepinephrine, and ephedrine) and antibiotics. Some drugs are oxygen sensitive (e.g., pilocarpine and physostigmine), so antioxidants and/or protective packaging are employed. Important OTC preparations are artificial tears, hypertonic solutions for increasing water content in the cornea, eye washes, and various combinations of vasoconstrictors, astringents, demulcents and emollients for relief of irritation and allergic conjunctivitis.

Nasal, Inhalant, and Otic Liquids

Nasal liquids are usually aqueous solutions administered as drops or as nasal sprays to treat local conditions in the nasal passages and to achieve systemic access. Common drugs in these solutions are ephedrine sulfate and naphazoline hydrochloride. They provide a sympathomimetic effect which reduces nasal congestion. Antibiotics, antihistamines and drugs for asthma prophylaxis are also used. Inhalants are vaporized to be carried into the respiratory system. In the traditional method, solutions of a drug are added to hot water and carried along with the steam produced. Alternatively, water can be vaporized by mechanical methods. Often the inhalant solution requires a nonaqueous solvent to dissolve the drug, an example being benzoin in alcohol.

Otic liquids intended for administration to the ear as drops encompass both solutions and suspensions. In addition to water, glycerin is often used to increase viscosity so that medication is held in the ear longer. Glycerin reduces tissue swelling and helps remove wax. Drugs intended for local action are analgesics (e.g., benzocaine), antibiotics (e.g., neomycin) and anti-inflammatory agents (e.g., cortisone).

Parenteral Preparations

Parenteral preparations are those that are administered by injection by the insertion of a needle under or through one or more layers of skin or mucous membranes. Such injections generally consist of a single dose of medication as contrasted to intravenous administration in which large volumes of fluid are infused continuously into the body over long periods. Early in this century it was proved that the chills and fever often experienced after intravenous injection were caused by pyrogens. This finding gave impetus to the development of the standards and technology in place today to achieve exceptional purity in this dosage form.

Solutions, emulsions and suspensions are used as parenteral preparations. Techniques used to make them are similar to those described above except for the extra attention required to attain high purity and sterility. Especially fine particle size for suspensions is required. Even so, suspensions cannot be used for intravenous injections since even the finest particles can block blood vessels. Variations of the physical state of the drug and the level of dispersion are used to control the rate of absorption of the drug into the bloodstream. As an example, injectable solutions of soluble, amorphous forms of insulin are quick acting, whereas suspensions of more crystalline forms, such as zinc-modified versions, are long acting due to their reduced solubility in tissue fluids. Mixtures are used to achieve a range of bioavailability.

A recent development in increasing the duration of drug bioavailability is the use of biodegradable polymers to encapsulate drugs in microparticulate suspensions. Examples of such applications are leuprolide acetate and goserelin acetate (for the treatment of prostate cancer) which are released at a declining rate over the course of a month after intramuscular or subcutaneous injection. In another development, ferric oxide has been added to coated particles so that antibiotics, for example, can be concentrated at a specific target area in the body by the use of an external electromagnetic field. Emulsions as vehicles for some drugs such as diazepam have been shown to have advantages of isotonicity, neutral pH, enhanced therapy and reduced toxicity [13].

IV Liquids

Liquids intended for administration by injection of large volumes through intravenous infusion are placed in a separate category from parenteral preparations because of their special requirements. The large volume of fluid introduced into the bloodstream provides unusual opportunity for even trace contaminants in the fluid to accumulate and reach toxic levels in the body. IV fluids are sterile solutions of simple chemicals such as sugars, amino acids, and electrolytes. They are used to replace body fluids and electrolytes, to promote tissue growth and repair and to provide either supplemental or total nutrition. For total parenteral nutrition, the admixture usually contains five components: protein source, calories, vitamins, electrolytes and trace elements. Calories are provided by dextrose and fat emulsions. Vitamins are often a combination of water soluble and oil moieties. Electrolytes commonly used include salts of sodium, potassium, calcium and magnesium. Trace elements include zinc, copper, manganese and chromium. IV fluids are also convenient vehicles for introducing drugs by adding them to the fluid during infusion or to the IV fluid prior to injection. Obviously, it is important to be sure that such mixtures are compatible, so that drug effectiveness is not compromised, and to be certain that undesirable precipitates are not produced.

Other Liquids

A douche is an aqueous solution used for cleansing or disinfecting the surface of the body or body cavities. Douches include those for cleansing the eye, throat, nasal passages and vagina. While some douches are supplied as liquids, more often the preparation is dispensed as a powder or tablet to be dispersed in water.

Enema preparations are administered into the rectum to facilitate evacuation of the bowel, to access the systemic route and to treat a localized condition topically. For evacuation of the bowel, typical solutions (sodium chloride, sodium bicarbonate, sodium monohydrogen phosphate, sodium dihydrogen phosphate and soap) are usually injected slowly using a syringe. A popular commercial preparation consists of a solution of mixed phosphates. An example of local treatment is a rectal enema containing sulfasalazine to treat ulcerative colitis. Solutions intended for systemic absorption contain such drugs as aminophylline to treat asthma and bronchospasm and the steroids, hydrocortisone and methylprednisolone acetate.

Gargles are aqueous solutions administered to the pharynx and nasopharynx and usually contain an antiseptic intended for local treatment only. Mouthwashes are similarly formulated and often used interchangeably with gargles. Typical anti-infective agents used include hexetidine, cetylpyridinium chloride and boric acid, all of which can be effective in reducing bacterial count and odors in the mouth. Cetylpyridinium chloride and dibucaine hydrochloric mouthwashes help relieve pain from ulcerative lesions. Mouthwashes containing carboxolone are effective in treating orofacial herpes.

Packaging Needs of Liquids

Physical containment is a greater problem with liquids than with solids. As liquid viscosity decreases, the risk of leakage increases. Physical mixtures such as suspensions and emulsions can become unstable and settle out or separate over time. High viscosity liquids like syrups can be difficult to pour, especially at low temperatures. Evaporation of solvent increases viscosity, causes variation in drug concentration and can lead to precipitation of some components, which changes both potency and composition.

Maintenance of sterility is essential for most liquid products. Drugs in solution that are sensitive to oxygen or other gases tend to be more reactive than in solid forms. Examples were given above for ophthalmic solutions. Another example is a calcium hydroxide topical solution that reacts with carbon dioxide.

Many liquids must be dispensed in reasonably controlled doses while minimizing contamination of the remaining product. The method of dispensing must accommodate the viscosity of the liquid. For ophthalmic liquids, dispensing must be as drops. For nasal and bronchial applications the preferred form is a mist. For some preparations, dose control must be precise.

For injectable and intravenous products, the strictest requirements for absence of contamination and retention of sterility apply; packaging materials must not be a source of contamination. Container transparency is essential to the detection of undesirable particulates, changes in color, etc. Where IV mixtures, solutions, or suspensions are made extemporaneously, means must be provided for convenient and thorough mixing in the package to minimize contamination and maintain sterility. To dispense injectable fluids, multiple introductions of a needle to withdraw contents are required in a way that eliminates the introduction of contaminants and achieves complete closure upon removal of the needle.

OINTMENTS

The official *USP* definition of an ointment encompasses all semisolid preparations. Since methods of preparation and packaging needs are common for the various kinds of semisolids, the *USP* definition will be used here as well. Thus, the ointment category includes:

- ointments — oleaginous bases
- creams — emulsion bases
- gels — network structures of suspended particles swollen by the liquid
- pastes — creams with high solids content

Preparation

While historically a number of other oleaginous bases have been used for ointments such as vegetable oils and animal fats, hydrocarbons are now almost exclusively employed. Hydrocarbons usually consist of petrolatum sometimes modified with waxes or liquid petrolatum, and liquid petrolatum gelled with polyethylene resin. Oleaginous based ointments are generally prepared by dispersing drugs into a small portion of the base followed by addition of the remaining base. Dispersion is accomplished in mills and/or mixers and the base is sometimes melted to facilitate the process. Water soluble bases are also used. These consist of waxy, higher molecular weight polyethylene glycols, blends of solid and liquid polyethylene glycols and aqueous solutions gelled with solutes such as cellulose derivatives.

The principles for formulating and preparing creams are the same as for liquid emulsions. Often the oil phase is heated to enhance mixing, a heated aqueous phase is added, and the emulsion is slowly cooled with agitation to sustain the dispersion. The oil phase of the emulsion base is usually petrolatum and/or liquid petrolatum combined with higher molecular weight alcohols. The water phase, which usually dominates, contains the emulsifier and preservatives.

Topical Ointments

The choice of the base for topical ointments depends on drug compatibility, whether local or systemic effects are desired, and user preferences. Petrolatum bases have no odor, no taste, a high degree of compatibility with medications such as antibiotics, a wide range of melting points and a tendency to increase skin hydration. The latter is important not only for skin moistening but also for enhancing the absorption of drugs such as steroids through the skin and into the circulatory system. Gelled mineral oils are sometimes substituted for petrolatum since they release drugs faster because of their more liquid structure. Despite these advantages, the vast majority of dermatologic drug preparations are formulated as a cream or emulsion because of the overwhelming disadvantage of oleaginous based ointments—greasiness and difficulty in removal. Water soluble gels overcome this disadvantage and can aid in the delivery of a drug, such as steroids, for which gels are especially formulated. However, enhanced bioavailability is not necessarily assured by the use of gels since such bases can dehydrate the stratum corneum and hinder absorption.

Allergic reactions and irritation can be a problem with ointments. Most commonly the cause is a component of the base. Irritation is usually tested by repeated application of both components and the complete formulation to the skin of a rabbit.

Ophthalmic Ointments

The advantage of ointments over liquids for ophthalmic applications is longer contact time in the eye with greater total drug bioavailability. The disadvantages of ointments are the somewhat greater dosage variability and interference with vision. Ophthalmic ointments must be prepared under the strictest conditions of purity and sterility, and antimicrobial agents are included in the formulation. To minimize tissue irritation, large particles must not be present and special care must be used to eliminate particulate contamination such as metal fragments. Typical bases used are mixtures of petrolatum and mineral oil, anhydrous lanolin or mineral oil gelled with polyethylene.

Packaging Needs

The main problem with ointments is the difficulty of administering these highly viscous products. Means must be provided if something more convenient and sanitary than using the finger is desired. Although exact control of dosage is rarely a requirement, there are instances where this is necessary. Some ointment ingredients are volatile and/or light sensitive.

For ophthalmic ointments, there is the critical need of achieving and maintaining purity and sterility. Where products are terminally sterilized, packages must be able to withstand sterilization conditions.

TRANSDERMAL SYSTEMS

As discussed in previous sections, drugs can be absorbed through the skin and into the bloodstream for systemic action. A systemic dosage form that is especially convenient and has broad flexibility in control of drug bioavailability is the transdermal system which is becoming increasingly popular. These systems are the familiar patches of scopolamine, nitroglycerin, estradiol, clonidine, and fentanyl. A patch is also available that provides day-long supplements of Vitamin C which is claimed to be superior to short lived oral dosages. In general, administration is limited to a fixed rate diffusion of low dosage, lipophilic, non-irritating drugs.

A transdermal patch is a thin, multilayered composite, shown in Figure 2.15. Typically it consists of a reservoir containing the drug preparation, an outside layer which serves to protect the ingredients from the environment, a skin-side layer that controls the rate of transfer of the drug into the skin and an adhesive layer to adhere the patch to the skin. In some cases, the patch is simply a top barrier layer containing an ointment which is in direct contact with the skin and contained by a ring of adhesive. Simpler yet, the drug can be dispersed in an adhesive layer carried by a barrier

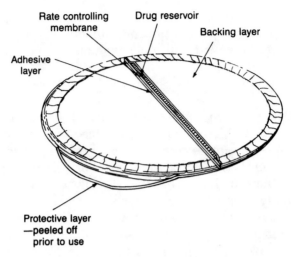

FIGURE 2.15. A transdermal patch.

layer. In each of these structures, a peelable strip is used to protect the adhesive side of the patch prior to use.

In patches where the liquid or semisolid preparation is in direct contact with the skin, the rate of drug absorption through the skin is determined by the factors previously described. In a variation of the direct contact approach, the medication is held in a sponge. However, when a membrane is interposed between the skin and the drug preparation, and when the rate of absorption of the preparation by skin is relatively rapid, the membrane is the rate-controlling element. Such membranes have a tailored permeability to the active drug which produces the desired absorption rate, resists solvents and can be bonded by heat or adhesives to facilitate fabrication of the patch. Ethylene vinyl acetate film is commonly used for the membrane. Polyurethane films, which are under development for this application, can be formulated with a broad range of permeabilities [14].

Also under development is an added diffusion enhancer and controller, iontophoresis, where a small electric current is used to propel drugs through the skin. Most drugs have the necessary charge to adequately respond to the current which is kept at a low enough level to avoid creating a tingling sensation. Miniaturized electronics and batteries are small enough to be included in a Band-aid sized patch. Systems would include both continuous and intermittent delivery [15].

A problem with transdermal systems is that users can be allergic to or their skin irritated by the drug or system components. The problem increases when patches are used for long periods or are repeatedly placed at the same location. Where the drug is at fault, the rate of drug release can be reduced as in the system for delivery of bupranolol, which irritates the skin at high release rates. In this case, a polyisobutylene adhesive with low permeability is chosen. Alternatively, the drug itself can be modified to be nonirritating. It is apparent that tests must be conducted on humans early in the development of potential transdermal systems [16].

Packaging Needs

Transdermal products often contain highly volatile ingredients and must be protected from loss by diffusion.

AEROSOLS

The *USP* defines pharmaceutical aerosols as "products that are packaged under pressure and contain therapeutically active ingredients that are released upon activation of an appropriate valve system" [17]. Traditionally, aerosols are regarded as a dosage form because of the formulation complexities imposed by the addition of compressed gases and liquids to the drug plus the specialized hardware required by the aerosol system. On the other hand, aerosols can be viewed simply as highly specialized packages that enable the convenient and controlled production of a spray mist of liquids or powders. This is the approach taken in Chapter Eight.

Preparation

While technically the term *aerosol* refers just to the mist of spray created by pressurized systems, it is commonly used to describe all products produced by release from a pressurized container, including foams and semisolids. The characteristics of these aerosol products depend on variations of the basic components of the system: the container, the propellant, the concentrate containing the active drug, the valve and the actuator. Propellants are compressed or liquified gases that exert a pressure consider-

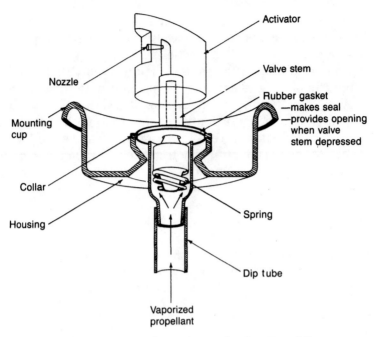

FIGURE 2.16. Aerosol actuator and valve assemblies.

ably in excess of atmospheric to provide the force required to expel the product. Liquified gases, either alone or in combination with cosolvents, also serve as a solvent for the active ingredients. Liquified gases include fluorochloro derivatives of methane and ethane as well as low molecular weight hydrocarbons such as butane and pentane. Compressed gases used include carbon dioxide, nitrogen and nitrous oxide. Often mixtures of propellants are employed to achieve an optimum pressure.

The combination of valve and actuator regulates and directs the flow of the contents [see Figure 2.16(a)]. The actuator is the button or spout on top of the aerosol container which is usually depressed to release the aerosol product. The design of the actuator (size of the orifice and the shape of the expansion chamber), in combination with the content formulation, determines the physical form of the discharge (spray mist, foam, wet stream or stream of powder) and the droplet size of a mist. Also, specialized designs permit discharge of product vertically, horizontally or at a 45-degree angle. For oral inhalation products, the adaptor allows mixing of the aerosol with air to attain the appropriate concentration and dispersion of fine droplets.

The valve is located immediately below the actuator and is opened by the action of the actuator stem. The valve is spring-loaded so that at rest it is closed and retains the pressurized aerosol contents. The size of the valve opening determines the rate of product delivery. For metered dosage delivery, the valve is expanded to include a chamber which is precharged with the aerosol product so that opening the valve discharges only the contents of the chamber. The valve housing is attached to a cup or ferrule whose edge is curled to mate with the opening in the aerosol can to permit attachment and seaming.

The propellant, either liquified or compressed gas, may simply provide the pressure to force liquid or semisolid preparations out through an activator or nozzle. Such an aerosol for a drug solution in water is shown in Figure 2.17. Here the drug solution and the propellant are immiscible and three phases are formed: the drug solution, the liquid propellant and the propellant gas. In this aerosol, the spray mist is formed entirely by the action of the actuator. However, if the propellant is dispersed in the discharging liquid, rapid evaporation of the propellant gas as the stream emerges from the actuator greatly enhances mist formation. One method of accomplishing this dispersion is to shake the contents prior to use but this only works if the propellant floats on top of the solution whereas normally, as shown in Figure 2.17, the liquid propellant rests on the bottom of the container. Thus, mixtures of water and alcohol for the solution and mixtures of propellants are chosen to achieve the slight density difference which is necessary for the liquified propellant to float on the solution.

Another method for dispersing the propellant in the drug solution is to feed the vaporized propellant separately to the actuator where it is mixed with a stream of the solution which is driven also by the pressure of the propellant. Since the stream of propellant is very rapid, a very fine, dry spray of small particles is produced with minimum use of propellant. These sprays do not produce the chilling effect of other aerosols.

The maximum effect on mist formation of evaporating propellant is achieved when the drug is soluble in the pure liquified propellant or mixtures of the propellant with cosolvents such as alcohol, propylene glycol and polyethylene glycol. Since many drugs can be dissolved in such propellant systems, this is the most popular aerosol for drug solutions. As shown in Figure 2.18, there are only two phases: the liquified and vaporized propellant solution. Another two phase system is also used which consists of a

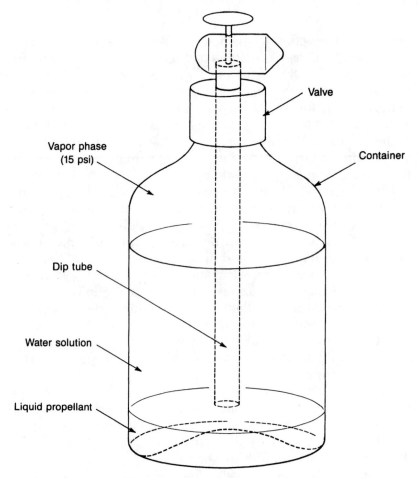

FIGURE 2.17. Three-phase aerosol.

stable suspension of the drug in the liquid propellant from which a spray of dry solid particles is created.

Foams are produced from emulsions when the liquified propellant is dispersed as the discontinuous phase in a continuous phase of the active ingredients, surfactants and other liquids. The dispersion is achieved by shaking the contents before use. Alternatively, foams can be produced with soluble gases such as carbon dioxide or nitrous oxide dissolved in an emulsion.

Several aerosol systems have been designed to isolate the solution or suspension from the liquified propellant. In one type, a plastic bag which contains the product is inside the aerosol container. The bag is surrounded by the propellant. When the valve is opened, the propellant squeezes the bag, forcing product out of the valve. This system is useful for dispensing liquids and ointments. In another approach, the propellant is maintained inside the container in a small, separate pressurized can. When the valve is activated, the propellant is released to form a venturi effect that draws product from a dip tube in the main container and mixes it into the propellant just prior to spray formation.

The general advantages of aerosols are that they are convenient and easy to use. Medication is readily available at the push of a button. Sterility is relatively easy to maintain during the life of the product.

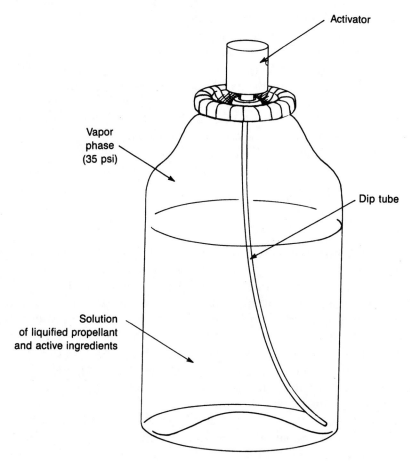

FIGURE 2.18. Two-phase aerosol.

Topical Aerosols

The application of a spray mist or foam over an inflamed part of the skin is much less irritating than applying liquids and ointments by physical contact. The cooling effect of liquified gas aerosols is also soothing. Another advantage is that a very thin, more economical coating can be applied, avoiding overuse of products. Driven by these advantages, a wide range of topical products are offered in aerosol form: local anesthetics (e.g., benzocaine, ethyl chloride and tetracaine); antiseptics (including antibiotics); germicides; first-aid and burn preparations (combining antiseptic and local anesthetics); spray-on protective films; dermatological preparations which contain steroids such as cortisone or prednisolone, antihistaminics, calamine, zinc oxide or sulfur; and foot medications containing undecylenic acid or its salts.

Many topical aerosols are based on solutions, but in some the active ingredients are suspended in the liquified propellant. This is usually the case for drugs like antibiotics and steroids which have limited solubility. The mist produced by these systems is a powder. Lubricants and other additives are employed to reduce caking, agglomeration and valve clogging, with surfactants aiding in dispersion stability. Foam aerosols are not widely used but have been suggested for rectal, vaginal and burn preparations.

Topical aerosols use hydrocarbon propellants. These carry with them a flammability potential that has been reduced by improved valve designs, but it is still significant.

Inhalant, Oral, and Nasal Aerosols

Inhalants are drugs intended to be vaporized and inhaled for quick relief of nasal and bronchial congestion. Traditionally, the vapors are produced by addition of the medication to hot water or by a mechanical device that produces a mist such as an atomizer. Aerosols can also be used with the drug dispersed in liquified gas and sprayed in an enclosed space to create a breathable medicated vapor. Alternatively, a handkerchief can be sprayed and held to the face for inhalation.

For access to the deeper recesses of the respiratory system, nebulizers and oral aerosols are used. Of the two, oral aerosols are more convenient with their self-contained pressure and ready-to-use contents in a small container. Metering valves allow automatic control of dosage levels. Because of the fine dispersion of solution droplets, therapeutic action is rapid. However, oral aerosols are complicated delivery systems that require the user to correctly perform a number of maneuvers during use to assure proper deposition of the drug in the respiratory airways. Furthermore, different products have significantly different directions for optimum effectiveness.

Despite their complications, oral aerosols are widely used for the symptomatic treatment of asthma and other bronchial ailments. In addition, they are used for systemic access, especially for drugs that degrade in the gastrointestinal tract. Finally, aerosols provide an alternative systemic route when oral or parenteral routes are inappropriate for the drug or when drugs that might be incompatible with the aerosol drug are already being given by these other routes. Both solution and suspension systems are used for inhalation applications. For suspensions, the critical need is for very fine particle size in the initial suspension along with steps to minimize agglomeration such as limiting the solubility of the drug in the propellant and minimizing the moisture content of the propellant. Surfactants and lubricants are also helpful in inhibiting agglomeration.

As an alternative to drops and sprays, nasal aerosols have been recently introduced that feature metered dosage, excellent depth of penetration into the nasal passages (avoiding inadvertent penetration into the lungs), small particle size, better maintenance of sterility, decreased mucosal irritation and greater flexibility in drug formulation. Two products currently available are suspension formulations containing dexamethasone sodium phosphate and beclomethasone dipropionate for the relief of nasal and hay fever symptoms. These products, when formulated for solution spray application, proved to be too irritating to nasal membranes because of large particles. Formulations for nasal aerosols are very similar to oral aerosols with the principal difference being the design of the adaptor.

Packaging Needs

Most importantly, aerosol containers must safely contain the propellant pressure. Most applications are low enough pressure so that the simple steel cans are practical. However, this limits the design of distinctive shapes, so aluminum containers are more often used to provide a wider variety of more functional and attractive designs. Stainless steel containers are used where high pressures are required. Where container interaction is a problem either glass or stainless steel is used. The use of plastic for aerosol containers is increasing. The pressure must be releasable in an easy, controlled fashion. For some medications such as inhalants, the release must be in automatically controlled dosages.

SUMMARY

The requirements that arise most often in these descriptions of packaging needs are product containment, product protection, product dispensing, and sterility. Product containment is more difficult for liquids and aerosols than solids. Product protection needs vary considerably and depend primarily on the chemistry of the drug rather than the dosage form. Liquids, semisolids and parenterals in particular require convenient product dispensing that is ideally an integral part of the package. Controlled dose dispensing is frequently desired or required for liquids and aerosols. The sterility requirement is probably the one most frequently cited for all the dosage forms.

The least demanding dosage forms are solids. Protection from moisture and physical damage are the main packaging requirements. At the other extreme, the most demanding dosage forms are ophthalmic, injectable and intravenous fluids where the highest standards of purity and sterility must be attained and preserved by the package which must also fulfill special dispensing needs.

REFERENCES

1. FDA. 1990. Title 21 of Code of Federal Regulations (CFR), Part 210 (April 1):74–95.
2. Gennaro, A. R., ed. 1990. *Remington's Pharmaceutical Sciences, 18th Edition.* Easton, PA: Mack Publishing Company, p. 1520.
3. Ibid., p. 1640.
4. Baes, E. A. 1981. *Manufacturing Chemist & Aerosol News* (March):33.

5. Jones, B. E. 1987. *Manufacturing Chemist* (January):27,29,31.

6. Maconachie, S. 1977. *Manufacturing Chemist and Aerosol News* (August):35.

7. Ebert, W. R. 1977. *Pharm. Tech.*, 1:44.

8. Astorri, E., G. Bianchi and G. La Cann. 1979. *J. Pharm. Sci.*, 68:104.

9. Arnold, J. D., J. Baldridge, B. Riley and G. Brody. 1977. *J. Clin. Pharmacology*, 15:230.

10. Yamahira, Y., T. Naguchi, H. Takenaka and T. Maeda. 1979. *Chem. Pharm. Bull.*, 27:1190.

11. Allen, L. V. 1990. *U.S. Pharmacist* (May):56–57.

12. Allen, L. V. 1990. *U.S. Pharmacist* (October):90–92.

13. Newton, D. W. 1991. *U.S. Pharmacist* (June):42–50.

14. Komerska, J. F. 1987. *J. Plastics and Sheeting*, 3(January):58–64.

15. Fisher, L. M. 1991. *New York Times* (May 26):F8.

16. Anon. 1990. *The Pharm. J.* (September 29):430–431.

17. *USP XXII*, p. 1689.

GENERAL REFERENCES

Gennaro, A. R., ed. 1990. *Remington's Pharmaceutical Sciences, 18th Edition.* Easton, PA: Mack Publishing Company.

King, R. E., ed. 1984. *Dispensing of Medication.* Philadelphia, PA: Mack Publishing Company.

Lachman, L., H. A. Lieberman and J. L. Kanig. 1986. *The Theory and Practice of Industrial Pharmacy, Third Edition.* Philadelphia, PA: Lea and Febiger.

CHAPTER THREE

The Regulatory Environment

Two federal agencies specifically regulate drug packaging: the Food and Drug Administration (FDA) and the Consumer Product Safety Commission (CPSC). Many acts of Congress also apply to drug manufacture and packaging: TOSCA, OSHA, Clean Air Act, RCRA, CERCLA (Comprehensive Environmental, Responsibility, Compensation, and Liability Act) but these apply broadly to the manufacture of other substances as well and will therefore not be discussed here. Chapter Seven, which covers closures, will deal with CPSC, so only the FDA and the U.S. Pharmacopoeia (USP) will be dealt with in this chapter—the USP because it establishes standards that the FDA uses as part of the regulatory process.

The regulatory process is very complex. It is summarized here solely to give the reader an understanding of the ways in which it affects packages and the packaging process. For the detailed understanding needed by anyone who engages in these processes, the original references must be consulted.

THE FOOD AND DRUG ADMINISTRATION

History of the FDA

The Food and Drug Administration was established by the Pure Food and Drugs Act of 1906 which was enacted because of increasing problems with adulterated foods, especially packaged meat. At the outset, the FDA was only authorized to police interstate commerce for adulterated or mislabeled food and drugs, not to issue regulations or standards to protect public health nor to engage in preclearance procedures.

In 1938, under the Federal Food, Drug and Cosmetic Act, the FDA was authorized to establish definitions and standards of identity for foods and to preclear new drugs after appropriate safety evaluations. This law also included regulation of cosmetics for possible misbranding and/or adulteration.

The growing use of food additives after World War II led to amendments in 1958 that covered food additives including substances that might transfer to foods from packaging materials or other food contact surfaces. An amendment in 1960 dealt specifically with food colorants.

In the wake of the discovery in 1962 that thalidomide could cause birth defects, the FDA was empowered to base preclearance of drugs on efficacy as well as safety *and* to use an affirmative clearance process rather than the waiting period/nonobjection procedure heretofore used.

Basically, the law now prohibits "the introduction, or the delivery for introduction, into interstate commerce any new drug, unless an approval of an application filed in accordance with the provisions of section 505(b) [of the 1938 Act] is effective with respect to such drug" [1]. Section 505(b) in its entirety states:

> Any person may file with the Secretary an application with respect to any drug subject to provisions of section 505(a). Such persons shall submit to the Secretary as part of the application (1) full reports of investigations which have been made to show whether or not such drug is safe for use and whether such drug is effective in use; (2) a full list of the articles used as components of such drug; (3) a full statement of the composition of such drug; (4) a full description of the methods used in, and the facilities and controls used for, the manufacture, processing, and packing of such drug; (5) such samples of such drug and of the articles used as components thereof as the Secretary may require; and (6) specimens of the labeling proposed to be used for such drug. [1]

To implement the law, the FDA has prepared and issued regulations which are published as part of Title 21 of the Code of Federal Regulations (CFR). They describe in detail the types and quantities of studies and attendant data that must be submitted for review and approval. The major regulations are contained in section 312, which covers investigational new drugs (IND), and section 314, which covers new drug applications (NDA).

In the early 1980s, the FDA began to issue guidelines and define procedures to clarify just how a manufacturer should go through the approval process. These procedural clarifications dealt separately with procedures for NDA, procedures for IND, and guidelines to manufacturers on application and testing formats. These guidelines concerned themselves, in separate sections, with the manufacture of drugs, samples and analytical data for methods validation, stability and packaging [2]. The packaging guideline was published in the *Federal Register* for comment on February 1, 1984 and was finalized three years later.

It is important to note that although there are a growing number of aids being published to take the strain out of reading CFRs and the *Federal Register*, the only official texts that the FDA will accept are the CFR, the *Federal Register*, and their explanatory booklets. If a commercially published aid leads the packager astray, too bad.

THE DRUG APPROVAL PROCESS — GENERAL

We will now discuss the approval process in summary form and then return in the next section to details of the packaging guidelines.

Packaging is considered part of the drug, so data on packaging must be submitted as part of the NDA. The regulations provide that the NDA application must include "full information . . . in sufficient detail to permit evaluation of the adequacy of the described methods of manufacture (including packaging) . . . and the described facilities and controls to determine and preserve the identity, strength, quality, and purity of the drug" [3]. They also require information "with respect to the characteristics of the test methods employed for the container, closure or other components of the drug package to assure their suitability for the intended use" [4]. Samples of the finished market packages for each dosage form of the drug must accompany the application [5].

The information required concerning the package is so detailed that it frequently involves information that the package manufacturer or his suppliers consider proprietary. To protect this kind of information from becoming publicly known, the FDA has established the Drug Master File (DMF). The proprietary information is submitted directly by the manufacturer to the FDA. It is kept in the DMF which can be accessed by the FDA only when authorized to do so by the NDA submitter. However, this is only background information; the drug manufacturer must also demonstrate that the proposed package will maintain the quality, purity, identity and strength of the drug.

A manufacturer who wants to change the package from one already approved will usually have to submit a supplemental application, particularly if the proposed change ". . . could alter the conditions of use, the labeling, the safety, effectiveness, identity, strength, quality or purity of the drug or the adequacy of the manufacturing methods, facilities, or controls to preserve them" [6]. When considering supplemental applications, the FDA focuses mainly on questions of stability. Some changes may require prior approval. Some may be made without prior approval but must be reported in annual reports to the FDA.

PACKAGING GUIDELINES

Guidelines issued in final form in 1987 present very specific recommendations as to the information that must be supplied in an IND or NDA about the package and its components. We have chosen not to reprint them in their entirety here but only to provide a flavor for the degree of detail that the FDA likes to have. (The guidelines in their entirety may be found, for example, in *Pharmaceutical Manufacturing*, June, 1984, pp. 32 ff.) The following summary description is adapted from Casola [1].

Chapter One of the guidelines begins by pointing out that USP supplies information about how many drugs should be packaged. It is essential to note that *if a drug is listed in the USP compendium*, it is considered misbranded if the packager does not follow those recommendations *unless* the packager receives explicit permission to deviate from them [7].

The next chapter of Guidelines deals with containers and closures. The section on containers covers four types: parenteral (ampules, vials, bottles, cartridges, prefilled syringes and bags); nonparenteral (bottles, unit dose and tubes); pressurized containers; and bulk containers.

Parenteral

For glass ampules and vials, the information required includes the manufacturer's name, the glass type, a physical description of the container, its chemical resistance, its light transmission if applicable, compatibility with the contents which includes leaching and/or migration tests, a sampling plan and acceptance specifications.

For plastic vials, the information required includes the name of the manufacturer; the plastic type; its composition (including the method of resin manufacture); the method of container manufacture with a full description of analytical controls; a physical description; the light transmission if applicable; certain USP tests (biological, physicochemical and permeation); vapor transmission data if applicable; additional toxicity tests not in *USP*; information on compatibility; and finally, the sampling plan and acceptance specifications.

The items needed for cartridges, prefilled syringes and large volume containers are the same as described above—if made of glass, under glass ampules; if made of plastic, under plastic vials.

The request for composition and method of manufacture of plastics is a very sensitive item for plastics companies, who originally resisted supplying this information. However, FDA remains adamant on this point because plastics manufacturers use many additives and there is always the possibility that they could be absorbed by the drug—a matter of great concern to the FDA.

Nonparenteral

The guidelines for glass and plastic bottles are very similar to those for glass and plastic parenteral containers except that a description of the desiccant, if present, is required and biological tests are not required. Strip and blister packages and tubes are covered by the same recommendations as plastic vials except that information should be presented on the adhesives used.

Pressurized Containers

For these, the guidelines emphasize information needed on the component parts of the valve closure and container plus information on the adequacy of the valve and activator for the intended use; proper leak-testing controls; leaching and migration tests, if applicable and information on compatibility.

Bulk Containers

Guidelines for this category are very similar to nonparenteral guidelines except that bulk containers used for temporary, short-term drug storage are exempt from the reporting requirement.

The last section of Chapter Two deals with closures: caps, liners, innerseals, and elastomeric stoppers used for parenteral vials. As discussed in later chapters of this book, closures are as important as the rest of the container, so the information required parallels that required for containers. Also included are information requirements that are logical and specific for closures: the seal mechanism used for caps, including torque data; a description of the innerseal, if used; special information required when an elastomeric closure is used; and special information about medicine droppers, if used.

Chapter Three, entitled Suitability of Package Components for Intended Use, deals mainly with plastics. The first section discusses the physical, chemical, and biological characteristics of plastic containers and explains the importance of a detailed elucidation of these characteristics relative to the use of a particular plastic container and/or closure for a particular drug.

The next section covers specifications and the tests that are needed to assure that each batch of plastic meets the specifications. Examples of tests suggested are IR spectroscopy, thermal analysis, melt viscosity, molecular weight, degree of crystallinity and film thickness. Biological testing is discussed, as are tests for elastomeric closures, i.e., integrity after multiple penetrations.

It is crucially important to note that the FDA will not accept compatibility tests that are not conducted in a real-life situation. The testing must be done on the actual container and closure containing the actual drug in question. For example, it is not sufficient simply to test the container material in standard test solutions to assess leaching and migration factors.

The adhesive and ink section of Chapter Three deals mainly

with tests to determine whether or not the organic components of these materials will migrate through plastic container walls or through elastomeric stoppers.

Chapter Four of the guidelines deals with IND applications. The container and closure to be used for a new drug in the investigational stage must be described for approval in the same detail as is needed for the final container. This allows for the fact that the container chosen for use during clinical trials may be quite different from the final container that will be used when the drug is commercial. In general, the FDA prefers that the containers used during the investigational process provide maximum protection and be as inert as possible; in other words, they prefer glass.

Chapter Five deals with changes in packaging for drugs already on the market. Generally, if a container change is contemplated, the packager must file for an amendment or submit a supplement and provide information on the proposed changes in:

- container type [a change of material (glass to plastic) or container style (bottle to blister package)]
- closures and/or liners
- the components of any plastic material used
- suppliers or fabricators
- packaging facilities

In cases where the packager uses polyethylene and proposes a change in resin supplier or a change from one type of HDPE or LDPE to another type of HDPE or LDPE, the FDA will allow such changes without prior approval, provided that the container/closure system originally adopted and the testing protocols for it have already been approved; it is demonstrated that the new container is equivalent to the old by use of tests described either in the NDA or in *USP*; and stability studies originally performed to establish the expiration date have been expanded to include the new container to be used.

This lengthy discussion of the scrutiny the FDA applies to drug packages and the comprehensive nature of the disclosures they require explains in part why drug packagers are reluctant to change an approved package and why they adopt changes so much more slowly than do food packagers.

CURRENT GOOD MANUFACTURING PRACTICES (CGMP)

Introduction

The CGMP described in this section were first established as regulations in 1938 by the FDA. The latest amendments were made in 1978. They are now contained in part 211 of 21 CFR, beginning on page seventy-six of the April, 1990, edition [10]. They cover every aspect of drug manufacture and are taken very seriously. Any drug manufactured or packaged in a way that does not conform to them is legally regarded as adulterated. However, the CGMP are quite general when it comes, for example, to materials selection. The FDA exerts control by insisting on maintenance of stability, strength, quality, purity, and efficacy; it's up to the packager to decide how to maintain these characteristics.

Summary of CGMP Applied to Packaging

The sections which bear on packaging are subpart E ("Control of Components and Drug Product Containers and Closures") and subpart G ("Packaging and Labeling Control"). In this discussion, the numbers appended refer to specific sections. These regulations and controls apply only to the drug manufacturing process and not to the ways in which a product is additionally labeled for advertising and display purposes.

Subpart E

Section 211.80 includes general requirements that deal with written procedures, storage and handling, and grouping of containers for identification.

211.82 covers receipt and storage of untested materials and components and procedures for grouping and examining these.

211.84 — testing and approval — deals with sampling, cleaning, opening, reclosing, record keeping and marking. The testing procedure regulations deal with testing for conformity with specifications, certificates from the manufacturer which may be used in lieu of testing, testing intervals, microscopic examination when necessary and release for use.

211.86 — use of approved components — covers stock rotation.

211.87 deals with the frequency with which approved components must be re-examined.

211.89 sets up a system to control rejected components.

211.94 deals with containers and closures and requires that these must not be reactive, additive or absorptive so as to alter safety, identity, quality, strength or purity beyond established requirements; that closure systems provide adequate protection against foreseeable external factors and that containers and closures must be clean and, when necessary, sterilized and processed to remove pyrogens.

Subpart G

211.122 covers materials examination and usage criteria and contains regulations for maintaining and following written procedures, examination of packaging and labeling materials, separate storage of labeling materials, destruction of obsolete labels, monitoring of printing devices and requires that gang printing of labels be minimized. (The mislabeling hazards attendant upon gang printing are described in Chapter Seven of this book.)

211.125 covers labeling issuance and requires:

- generally strict control over labeling
- careful examination of labels issued for a particular batch
- procedures to monitor discrepancies
- destruction of excess labels bearing specific lot or control numbers
- storage procedures for returned labels
- maintenance of written procedures

211.130 deals with packaging and labeling operations and covers written procedures, avoidance of mixups, identifying each product by lot or control number, examination and inspection of equipment, the general setup before beginning operations and the documentation required for all of these matters.

211.132, entitled "Tamper Resistant Packaging for OTC Human Drug Products," requires that:

- All OTC drugs (except dermatological, dentifrice, insulin or throat lozenge products) must be packaged in a tamper resistant package.
- The package must have at least one barrier to entry which if breached will provide a reasonable indication that this has happened.
- The package must be distinctive by design, i.e., hard to reproduce (such as an aerosol container) or bear some identifying characteristic(s) that will be hard to reproduce.
- Two-piece hard gelatin capsules must have at least two tamper evident features unless sealed by tamper evident technology.
- The package must have a prominent statement to tell consumers what the tamper evident feature is and placed so that it is unaffected if the package is tampered with.

211.134 deals with inspection of products during finishing operations to be sure they are correctly labeled and that a final visual examination of a sample of finished product is performed for additional confirmation of correct labeling. As discussed in Chapter Seven, the FDA prefers, but does not require, 100% inspection for labeling accuracy.

211.137 requires that each drug product bear an expiration date on the label. Exempt from this are OTC products if their labels do not bear dosage limitations and if they have been shown to be stable for at least three years. Examples of such products are medicated shampoos, topical lotions, medicated toothpaste, various creams and ointments and rubbing alcohol. All of these are "acceptable for frequent and often prolonged use without dosage limitation, and typically the contents of the retail package are used in a relatively short period of time."

Useful review articles that elaborate on the packaging aspects of the expiration date regulations have appeared [8]. The referenced article was written by an FDA official, who makes the following points:

- Expiration date data developed in plastic containers for solid dosage forms are transferable to glass containers without additional testing. For liquid dosage forms, this is not the case because the alkaline character of glass may alter the pH of the product and possibly its functionality.

- Closure changes do not need additional stability studies if the same innerseal or cap liner is used in the new system.
- Stability tests should always be performed on the smallest container size to be used. Tests on the largest size will then reveal whether intermediate sizes must also be tested.
- To encourage repackaging in unit dose containers, the FDA allows the use of a six-month expiration date without any testing so long as the package meets USP specifications for a Type B container (not to exceed 5 mg/day moisture penetration rate). Six months must be less than one-fourth of the unexpired time stated on the original container.

OTHER PACKAGING-RELATED REGULATIONS IN CFR

Insulin

21 CFR 429 covers drugs composed wholly or partly of insulin. Its packaging subpart, 429.10, requires that each batch be packaged in primary containers of sterile colorless transparent glass closed so that successive doses can be withdrawn with a hypodermic needle without removing the closure or destroying its effectiveness. The shape of the containers is specified in detail.

429.11 requires that the insulin container labels and inserts provide an incredible amount of detailed information:

- batch mark, potency, expiration date and storage requirements
- warnings about diabetes mellitus treatments
- description of volume markings
- how to sterilize the needle, withdraw the dose and clean the injection site
- notice that injection must be subcutaneous, not intramuscular or intravenous
- an explanation of hypoglycemia and the significance of sugar in the urine
- cautions about using the drug if it doesn't meet certain visual standards

and on and on for two more pages!

Insulin labels and containers or wrappers must be color coded to distinguish doses of different potencies and to distinguish between six or seven different types of insulin available for injection (globulin zinc insulin, isophane insulin suspension, insulin zinc suspension, protamine zinc insulin suspension, etc.).

Packaging Antibiotics

21 CFR 432 deals with the packaging and labeling of antibiotics. It stipulates that the container preserve the strength, quality and purity of the drug, and, using USP designations, be "tight" (or "well closed" for ointments and creams). The discussion includes sterile preparations, those designed for parenteral use and solid dosage forms such as tablets, capsules and suppositories, but no requirements are presented other than those in USP.

The labeling requirements are no different than those already covered in detail in the CGMP except for a long discourse on expiration dates which adds nothing substantive to the material appearing in earlier parts.

21 CFR 1.31 deals with label content in situations where the consumer is being offered "savings" by the manufacturer. Specifically, it covers the situation where a claim is made by the packager that the product is being offered at a lower price because of the container size or the quantity sold—the "large-economy-size" approach. In this situation, the packager must:

- offer the product in at least one other package size or labeled form
- restrict the economy claim to one package size
- offer a price lower by at least 5% than the other package sizes of the same drug
- show by records that the wholesale price was reduced enough to allow the retailer to meet the 5% discount without losing any of his normal markup

This part then goes to the deal with "cents off" situations, requiring, in summary, that:

- A regular selling price must have already been established.
- The price at all levels of distribution must be reduced by an equivalent amount.
- Records must show that the price to the retailer has been

reduced enough to allow him to offer the discount as above.

- The label must clearly show the regular price to which the discounted price applies.
- Shipments to the geographic area where the discount is offered must not exceed a 50% increase from the level of prior shipments to that area.

It then proceeds to deal with "introductory offers" in the same sort of way, with the clear intent of protecting the consumer against false claims of lower prices or economy packaging.

Drugs, foods, cosmetics and medical devices are covered under this sweeping control over unfair marketing practices. Although this material only marginally relates to packaging, it is cited here as another example of the surveillance maintained by the agency over drug manufacturers.

21 CFR 1302 regulates the packaging of controlled substances. The regulations deal only with special labeling requirements and not with container materials or design, with the exception that a tamper resistant feature must be incorporated.

21 CFR 610.61 and .62 deal with general biological products (blood products, vaccines, toxoids, toxins). The requirements deal only with the labeling of these products, albeit in some detail. For example, whole paragraphs are devoted to label position, label prominence and typefaces used.

VALIDATION

In recent years, the concept of validation has assumed increasing importance at the FDA and at the companies that manufacture and package drugs. Simply put, validation means answering this question: "Is this machine/process doing what it is supposed to do?" The FDA defines validation more formally and comprehensively as ". . . establishing documented evidence which provides a high degree of assurance that a specific process will consistently produce a product meeting its predetermined specifications and quality attributes" [9].

Validation in some form or another has been a part of manufacturing since the industrial revolution began, but only recently have government agencies been involved in the process. In the U.S., the birth of the nuclear power industry, with its awesome potential for catastrophic damage in the event of an accident, led at the beginning to extensive government regulation and mandatory scrutiny of equipment to ensure proper operation. A decade or so later, the FDA adopted a similar philosophy and codified it in the CGMP [10] and in the supplementary *Guidelines* [11] as one tool for protecting the public from the possibly lethal effects of incorrect procedures in drug manufacturing.

The scope of the processes that must be validated is very broad. Drug manufacturers interpret the regulations to mean that they must examine every process, every piece of equipment, and every procedure that impacts their product to be sure that the equipment, process, or procedure is doing what it is supposed to be doing and maintain written records of such examinations. The FDA suggests that the scope would probably include ". . . component specifications, air and water handling systems, environmental controls, equipment functions, and process control operations" [12]. For example, in the packaging of sterile pharmaceuticals, the manufacturer must validate, among other things, bottle and closure washers, fillers, cappers and labelers; water, air and vacuum supply systems; and the cleanliness of the room, the operators and their garments. More generally, validators of packaging processes must look systematically at every element of every packaging line that has any impact on the product and devise ways to prove that all these elements are doing what they are supposed to do. Careful and complete records must be kept on these activities—if there is no record, the FDA takes the position that validation never took place.

Validation of a machine or operation is carried out in an orderly sequence that begins with installation qualification. This involves first setting specifications on the machine that is purchased or built to carry out a specific operation. When that machine is installed, it is then tested to confirm that it performs as specified and to determine what its operating limits are. Before the machine is used in regular operations, a set of written procedures is prepared that tells the operator how to operate the machine and what the limits of the operation, such as speed, must be. Periodically, the machine is revalidated by challenge. A label position verifier, for example, can be challenged by deliberately adding unlabeled bottles to the inspection line. If the device does not reject all those bottles, it has failed the challenge.

Installation qualification is followed by performance qualification, a procedure which involves rigorous testing of each process to demonstrate the effectiveness and reproducibility of that process. The FDA emphasizes that when a process is being challenged to assess its adequacy, it is important that the challenge conditions simulate those that will be encountered during actual production, including so-called worst-case conditions [13].

Revalidation should be considered whenever there are changes in ". . . packaging, formulation, equipment, or processes which could impact on product effectiveness or product characteristics, and whenever there are changes in product characteristics" [14]. Importantly in packaging situations, any change in a material supplier should trigger the question, "Should we revalidate?" It is essential, of course, that what might be called a *philosophy* of revalidation be established, so that the necessity for revalidation in any particular case can be derived from that philosophy and so that the FDA inspector will be satisfied that revalidation is carried out in some systematic, rather than haphazard, fashion.

Although a major reason for drug manufacturers to spend millions of dollars every year on validation is FDA and CGMP requirements, the effort provides other benefits as well: insulation against product liability suits, reassurance of product efficacy, improvements in manufacturing yields and reductions in manufacturing costs which always accompany improvements in process and product quality ("make it right the first time") [15].

Pharmaceutical manufacturers began validation many years ago by focussing on the drug preparation and formulation segments of their operations. More recently they have concentrated on the packaging segment. For obvious reasons, the packaging of injectable fluids received early attention, but now all packaging, including OTC products, is subject to scrutiny. Thus every packaging process described in this book is subject to validation. Since a complete description of all the procedures involved in validating every drug packaging process would be beyond the intended scope of this work, we shall attempt by the exposition of principles and selected examples to give the reader some understanding of this subject, which has been described as "more an art than a science."

THE *U.S. PHARMACOPOEIA*

Introduction

The *U.S. Pharmacopoeia and National Formulary* is published by the U.S. Pharmacopoeial Convention. Every five years, the Convention brings out updates of this compendium and its supplements. By so doing, the Convention fulfills its primary purpose, which is ". . . to provide authoritative standards and specifications for materials and substances and their preparations that are used in the practice of the healing arts; [to] establish titles, definitions, descriptions, and standards for identity, quality, strength, purity, packaging and labeling, and also, where practicable, bioavailability, stability, procedures for proper handling and storage [of these materials]" [16]. Convention membership is drawn from the medical and pharmaceutical professions, educational institutions, professional and scientific organizations, and the Federal government.

The USP-NF includes all and only drugs "of established merit." Originally USP concerned itself solely with drugs while NF dealt with drug ingredients, but in 1974, both classes of materials were put in one volume.

When the first Pure Food and Drug Act was enacted in 1906, the USP had been in existence for almost ninety years. Congress wisely chose to recognize this expertise by designating the USP as the authority on standards for drug strength, quality, purity, and packaging. Thus from the beginning of the regulatory era, USP's guidelines and recommendations have had the force of law. To make this unmistakably clear, the law empowers governmental agencies, principally the FDA, to enforce the relevant laws

> . . . using certain defined aspects of the Compendia. Most commonly recognized are USP-NF standards for determining the identity, strength, quality, and purity of the articles and specifications for packaging and handling. In addition, many statutes and regulations . . . reference USP and NF requirements for packaging and storage of drugs. [17]

DRUG PACKAGING IN USP

USP concerns itself with two major elements of the drug packaging process: test procedures and container characteristics. There are five sections that deal with test procedures.

Test Procedures and Requirements

Section 1. This contains detailed descriptions of standards and tests for containers. The following items are included:

- tests for light transmission that must be passed for a container to meet USP's "light resistant" standard
- tests for resistance of glass containers to attack by water, the results of which enable the glass type to be classified as I, II, or III
- biological tests that enable plastic containers to be properly classified
- tests to determine the amount of water-extractable materials in plastics and the heavy metal content of the extracted residue
- special tests for ophthalmic containers
- tests for polyethylene containers to establish that they are polyethylene and are interchangeable
- requirements for expiration date labeling of drugs repackaged from bulk containers to unit dose containers
- labeling and packaging requirements for customized patient medication packages that contain two or more separate medications
- Permeation tests that establish how impermeable a container and closure must be in order to meet the standards for "tight" and "well-closed" containers. Generally speaking, a well-closed container protects the contents from extraneous solids and from loss of drug under ordinary conditions of handling, shipment, storage, and distribution. A tight container protects the contents from contamination by extraneous liquids, solids, or vapors, from loss of drug, and from efflorescence, deliquescence, or evaporation and is capable of tight reclosure [18]. These terms are used as packaging standards for most of the drugs that are included in individual monographs in *USP*. A separate section is devoted to unit dose containers that require different permeation test procedures.

It is noteworthy that the permeation tests and the permeation limits set for tight and well-closed containers in *USP* apply only to water vapor and not to oxygen or CO_2. Test procedures for these two gases are more complex than those for water vapor. Even so, this is clear evidence that most drug products, particularly solids, have far less sensitivity to oxygen than do packaged foods.

Section 2. This contains pertinent parts of the CGMPs which have already been described in detail above [19].

Section 3. This is a description of the requirements of the Poison Prevention Act which will be covered in Chapter Six of this book [13].

Section 4. This provides information on product stability and a general description of a comprehensive product stability program covering the five major stability categories:

- retention of chemical integrity and labeled potency
- retention of appearance, palatability, uniformity, dissolution, and suspendability
- retention of sterility or resistance to microbial growth
- retention of therapeutic effect
- no increase in toxicity

All of these items are dependent to a greater or lesser degree on the package material and design.

Section 4 also discusses the responsibility of the pharmacist to follow certain procedures when repackaging drugs to ensure retention of stability. This general advice deals mainly with care in selection of materials, labeling to caution the *purchaser* about appropriate storage conditions and providing the correct expiration date. It concentrates mainly on unit dose repackaging, emphasizing materials and labeling so that lot numbers and the correct expiration dates are included, proper records are kept and that safety closures, if required, are used [21].

Section 5. This general section on standards for special drug release systems includes a subsection on standards for the drug release characteristics of transdermal drug delivery systems [22].

Individual Drug Monographs

More than 1500 drugs and drug ingredients are described in the monograph section of *USP XXII*. For each drug, functional standards are set for the package and its label. The material standards are general in nature, leaving the packager latitude in choice of materials and package design. In some cases, glass is specified, but far more often, permeation is regulated by using terms such as "tight" or "well-closed," allowing the packager to use plastics if they meet the functional requirement. The labeling requirements, on the other hand, are generally quite specific, often specifying the wording that must be used. In the case of nitroglycerin, for example, the label must say: "Warning: to prevent loss of potency, keep these tablets in the original container or in a supplemental Nitroglycerin container specifically labeled as being suitable for Nitroglycerin tablets. Close tightly immediately after each use" [23].

In addition to these material and labeling standards, many other elements of the package are also covered in the monographs:

- To minimize accidental overdosing, IV injections are limited to one liter per container and colored and flavored aspirin tablets of 81 mg or less are limited to 36 tablets per container.
- Flavors and colors are prohibited in higher strength aspirin in the hope that tasteless white tablets will be less attractive to children.
- Multiple dose parenteral vials must contain an antimicrobial agent and the volume must be limited to 30 ml to prevent the patient from taking an overdose of this agent.
- Preparations for intraspinal, intracisternal or peridural administration must be packaged in single dose containers because of the doubtful safety of antimicrobial agents administered by these routes.
- All drug dosage forms covered in *USP* must have expiration dates put on by the manufacturer.
- Labels on injectable liquid containers must be placed so the liquid can be observed from top to bottom, so it can be swirled and judged for degree of particulate matter as well as color and fill [24].

Chapter Eight of this book incorporates these USP monograph requirements in its description of how individual drugs are packaged.

REFERENCES

1. Casola, A. R. 1988. "FDA's Guidelines on Pharmaceutical Packaging," presented at *ISPE/SPHE Joint Conference on Packaging, Kansas City, MO,* June 14, p. 2.

2. Ibid., p. 3.

3. FDA. 1984. Title 21 of the Code of Federal Regulations (CFR), 314.1 (c)(8).

4. Ibid., (c)(8)(i).

5. Ibid., (c)(9)(ii).

6. Kumkumian, C. S. 1976. "New Drug Applications Packaging Requirements," presented at *Packaging Institute Seminar, Anaheim, CA, September 23.*

7. 1982. Federal Drug and Cosmetic Act, section 502(g), 21 USC, section 352.

8. Davis, J. S. 1984. "GMP Aspects of Stability Programs," *Drug Devel. and Ind. Pharm.,* 10:1549.

9. FDA, Center for Drug Evaluation and Research. May, 1987. *Guidelines on General Principles of Process Validation,* p. 4.

10. FDA. 1990. Title 21 of the Code of Federal Regulations (CFR), 211.100.

11. *Guidelines,* op. cit. Reference [9].

12. Ibid., p. 11.

13. Ibid., p. 18.

14. Ibid., p. 21.

15. Hudson, B. J. and Simmons, L. 1992. "Validation of Package Seal Integrity," *Proceedings of Conference on Validation of Pharmaceutical Packaging,* Avalon Communications, P.O. Box 505, Southampton, PA 18966.

16. 1989. *USP XXII,* p. xxi.

17. Ibid., p. xlvii.

18. Zapotocky, J. A. 1976. "Understanding and Complying with *USP* Packaging Standards," *IOPP Packaging Report,* T-7611.

19. 1989. *USP XXII,* pp. 1675–1678.

20. Ibid., pp. 1685–1687.

21. Ibid., pp. 1703–1705.

22. Ibid., pp. 1581–1583.

23. Ibid., p. 953.

24. Heller, W. M. 1979. *Drug Intell. and Clin. Pharm.,* 13(April):225.

CHAPTER FOUR

Drug Packaging Materials

This chapter will cover the four main classes of materials used in primary drug packages: glass, metal, plastics and elastomers. We will discuss how these materials are made and their salient characteristics. Paper, a widely used packaging material, will not be covered, because it is almost never used as the sole component of the primary package. Its only application in the primary package is as one component of labels and of multilayer blister packages. We have also chosen not to discuss the once-popular cellulosic films because they have been almost completely replaced by plastics in drug packaging applications.

GLASS

Glass, originally the most widely used drug packaging material, is still favored for many drug packages because of its transparency, its excellent resistance to attack by most liquids and its total impermeability to gases.

Composition and Manufacture

Glass is made by melting, at temperatures as high as 1550°C, a mixture of inorganic oxides, mainly SiO_2, and alkali and alkaline earth oxides (fluxing oxides) which lower the melting point of the mix, making it easier to fabricate. As an alternative to these fluxing oxides, B_2O_3 can be used to reduce melt viscosity for fabrication purposes. Boron-containing glass has a higher melting point and a lower coefficient of thermal expansion, making it more durable and heat-resistant. It is also more inert since it does not contain the leachable oxides of alkali and alkaline earth metals.

When cooled, molten glass solidifies without crystallizing, forming an amorphous structure that is clear. Stabilizers of PbO_2 or Al_2O_3 are added to help prevent devitrification, the slow room-temperature crystallization process that gradually reduces clarity.

Glass is colored by adding iron oxides, MnO_2 and sulfur to produce an amber tint which excludes all light at wavelengths below 450 μm, or oxides of cobalt or chromium to produce shades such as blue and green, or selenium to produce a ruby color.

Three types of glass are used for drug containers. These are classified by USP as follows.

Type I

Type I glass is borosilicate glass containing about 80% SiO_2 and 10% B_2O_3 with smaller amounts of Al_2O_3 and Na_2O. This glass is the most inert and has the lowest coefficient of thermal expansion. Thus it is least likely to crack when subjected to a sudden temperature differential. It is commonly used in the manufacture of ampules and vials for parenterals.

Type I glass is preferred for solutions which can dissolve basic oxides, causing an increase in pH which would alter the efficacy or potency of the drug.

Type II

Type II glass is de-alkalized soda-lime glass with higher levels of Na_2O (13–17%) and CaO (5–11%). It is less resistant to leaching than Type I but more resistant than Type III. Type II glass, and the other types as well, can be made more resistant to leaching by treating the surface with SO_2 which converts surface oxides to soluble salts which can then be washed off with water. This surface treatment is effective for containers that are used only once but less so for containers that are repeatedly exposed to heat (as in repeated sterilization) that causes leachable oxides to diffuse to the surface of the container.

Type II glass has a lower melting point than Type I and is thus easier to fabricate. It also has a higher coefficient of thermal expansion. It is suitable for drug solutions that can be buffered to maintain their pH below 7, since labile oxides are more rapidly leached out by solutions of higher pH.

Type III

Type III glass has sodium and calcium oxide levels like Type II but contains more leachable oxides of other elements. Because of its relatively high reactivity, it is used only for anhydrous liquids and dry products.

Glass as a Drug Packaging Material

Glass has many advantages:

- It is totally impermeable to all gaseous environmental contaminants and to loss of essential volatile ingredients by diffusion through the container walls.
- It has excellent clarity and an attractive sparkle.
- It is easy to clean and sterilize with heat.
- Some glass types are the most inert of all drug packaging materials, being highly resistant to attack by all liquids except HF and strong caustic.
- It can be fabricated to produce a variety of shapes and can accept a wide variety of closure types.
- It is "filling-friendly," i.e., glass containers are easily unscrambled, filled, closed, labeled, and cartoned.
- Its good compressional strength allows cartons of glass containers to be stacked high in warehouses.
- Glass containers are easily hot-filled.

Glass also has some major disadvantages when compared to metals and plastics:

- With a density of 2–2.5 g/cc and a brittle character that requires thick container walls for adequate durability, glass containers are several fold heavier than their plastic (and even some metal) counterparts.
- When it breaks, glass shatters into numerous sharp fragments. Thus even when a glass container is deliberately and carefully broken, as when an ampule is opened, there is always the danger that glass fragments will be injected along with the drug.
- Because they are much heavier and sometimes more costly to fabricate than plastic containers, glass containers are more expensive.

Glass containers are now used for drug packaging in situations where inertness and perfect barrier are paramount considerations. They have been displaced by plastic containers in most drug packaging applications because plastic containers are lower in cost, weigh much less and are shatterproof.

METAL

The only metals used in primary drug packaging are tinplate and aluminum. The poor corrosion resistance of uncoated steel limits its use to galvanized or plastic-lined drums for bulk products.

Tinplate

Tinplate is made by applying a tin coating to sheet steel by electroplating or, less often, by dipping in molten tin. The thickness of a typical electroplated tin coating is less than 0.1 mil. After electroplating, the coating is flash-melted to produce a shiny surface. The tin coating improves corrosion resistance and facilitates joining by soldering. Since it is extremely thin, it usually has pinholes and so is usually overcoated with lacquers or enamels based on various polymers: acrylic, alkyd, vinyl, polyester or epoxy. Polymer coatings are applied after the container forming step to avoid exposing them to soldering temperatures. Tinplate finds its principal application in drug packaging as the material of construction for aerosol cans.

Aluminum

Aluminum is produced by the electrolysis of bauxite. The molten metal product of this process is cast into ingots to which small amounts of alloying metals (iron, copper, manganese) or silicon are added to increase strength. Cast ingots are then hot and cold rolled to strips about 10 mils thick for forming into rigid containers, 3–5 mils thick for semirigid foil containers, 1 mil thick for blister constructions and 0.3 mils thick for foil used in laminates to provide a gas barrier.

Aluminum work hardens when it is rolled but can be softened

by annealing. Unannealed (hard) foil is used in blister packages where its brittleness facilitates package entry. Annealed (soft) foil is used in barrier laminations because it tends to have fewer pinholes than hard foil.

Pinholes are formed during the foil rolling operation as the thickness is reduced below 1 mil. Oxide particles on the surface form weak spots when they are rolled into the foil. During subsequent rolling the metal tears away from these spots. Typically there are about 200 pinholes/m² which have a total area of only .00004 square inches in 100 square inches of foil. Because of these pinholes, foil below 1 mil is not a perfect barrier, but the adverse effect of pinholes is ameliorated to a great degree by laminating the foil to a plastic such as polyethylene—this is the form in which foil thinner than 1 mil is usually used [1].

Metals as Drug Packaging Materials

Aluminum and tinplate have many advantages and disadvantages in common:

- Both are strong and shatterproof, making them the materials of choice for aerosol containers.
- Both are totally impermeable to gases.
- As tube materials, both are flexible and have excellent deadfold characteristics. Even so, the lower reactivity and lower cost of plastic laminates are forcing metals, mainly aluminum, out of this application.
- The strength and deadfold character of metals make them the only practical material for use as the overcap on vials closed with an elastomeric stopper.
- Certain container shapes, such as cylinders, are readily fabricated from metals, but overall, both these metals must be classified less fabricable than plastic, particularly for complex shapes achievable only by processes such as blow molding.
- Both metals are easily decorated with very attractive finishes.
- Metals can provide the ultimate in tamper evidence for drug containers. This potential has not been tapped for a variety of reasons, principally economic, but remains a possibility if tampering ever becomes an acute problem.

- Both are naturally opaque, which can be either advantageous or disadvantageous.
- Both conduct heat well. In general, metals conduct heat about 100 times better than glass and 400 times better than plastics. This facilitates heat sterilization of package contents.

Tinplate has several disadvantages when compared to aluminum:

- It is more reactive and must be rendered unreactive with coatings which adds to cost. Aluminum is less reactive but still more so than glass and many plastics.
- Although metals are denser than glass, their strength and ductility allow the fabrication of containers with thinner walls than is possible with glass. Thus aluminum containers, with a density of about 2.7, can be much lighter than their glass counterparts and approach the light weight of plastic containers. Tinplate at a density of over 8 does not compete well in this contest.
- The lower density of aluminum means that aluminum containers are lower cost than those made of tinplate.

Ultimately, metals will be used only for aerosols, where strength and ductility make them the safest container, and as foil in laminates for blister and strip packaging and in other composite structures such as innerseal membranes and cap liners that require a barrier component. Plastics will drive metals out of all other drug packaging applications, primarily because of cost. The inherently higher cost of metal containers stems directly from their higher energy content. For example, about 20,000 BTUs are required to make a pound of plastic film, while 50,000 to 100,000 BTUs are consumed in making a pound of metal strip or foil [19]. When the eightfold density difference favoring plastics is factored in, the enormous per-container energy advantage of plastics becomes evident.

PLASTICS

Plastics are the fastest growing packaging material for food, drugs, and countless other products. In drug packaging as in other product categories, plastics are steadily replacing more traditional materials. The rate at which this replacement process is taking place is slower in drug packaging than for other products. There are good reasons for this.

First, the adverse health consequences of a drug being incorrectly packaged are greater than for most other products. Second, food processors concentrate far more intensively on packaging cost and packaging innovation than do drug manufacturers. As a result, the pace of change in drug packaging, as noted in Chapter One, is less than in food packaging.

Nevertheless, in most drug package categories, plastics now dominate:

- Seventy-five percent of the bottles used for oral solid dosage forms are plastic, and of these, about 80% are made of high density polyethylene.
- Eighty percent of the bottles for OTC liquids and 50% of the bottles for prescription liquids are plastic.
- Ninety percent of the ointment tubes are made of plastic or multilayer structures based on plastic.
- Almost all bottle closures are made of plastic, increasingly of thermoplastics such as polypropylene, and many of the rubber stoppers used for parenteral vials have been replaced by synthetic elastomers whose molecular structure and method of manufacture are closely akin to plastics.
- Pouches, bags, blister packs, and strip packs are either 100% plastic or are laminations consisting mainly of plastic.

In summary, it is safe to say that plastics are now the most widely used drug packaging material—metal aerosol cans and glass parenteral vials are the only important areas where plastics do not (and may never) dominate.

Plastics as Drug Packaging Materials

The dominant position of plastics in drug packaging results from several major inherent advantages that plastics have over glass and metal.

1. The density of plastics is 1–1.5 g/cc vs. glass at 2–2.5, aluminum at 2.7 and tinplate at 8.5. Thus plastic containers, particularly those made from plastic film, are many times lighter than those made of glass or metal. A lightweight container is less expensive to manufacture because it contains less raw material than a heavier one. As a result, rigid plastic containers are at least 20% lower in cost than their least expensive glass equivalents and the very lightweight flexible plastic containers are several fold lower in cost. This cost advantage, magnified by the lower freight costs enjoyed by lighter plastic containers, is the major reason for plastics' dominance in the packaging world.

2. A lightweight package is easier for consumers to handle: lifting, carrying and dispensing are all simplified.

3. Plastics have no rival in the ease with which complex container configurations can be manufactured. This allows designers the freedom to create shapes and styles that incorporate built in administration aids such as squeeze bottles, droppers, etc.

4. Closely related to design freedom is a unique option that plastics offer the designer: using thin flexible films to create the ultimate in lightweight, low cost packages.

5. Like metal and unlike glass, plastic containers are shatterproof. This is a major advantage for drug containers which are often handled in the bathroom environment over tile floors and countertops that can be fatal to a glass container dropped from wet hands.

6. Like glass and unlike metal, plastics can be crystal clear or totally opaque. This combination of safety (#5) and transparency is offered only by plastics.

7. Heat sealing, particularly of plastic films, provides an easily opened hermetic closure at lower cost than the hazardous fused glass closures or the soldered metal seams which require a tool to open them.

8. Plastics can be readily treated to accept printing inks and can be easily metallized; from the graphics standpoint, they are superior to glass or metals.

9. Aluminum is the only competitive drug packaging material that is produced in film form. However, aluminum foil is much more expensive than plastic film and is inferior in

toughness and strength. Foil is used in packaging drugs to provide a gas barrier, but coated plastic films can provide an equally effective barrier at lower cost.

Plastics have some drawbacks which limit their penetration of the drug packaging market.

1. No packaging material can match Type I glass for chemical inertness, and no plastic packaging material can match it for gas impermeability [2]. Although plastics of the fluorocarbon family are more inert than glass, they are too expensive to be used in packaging. As a practical matter, however, the inertness and gas barrier of lower cost plastics is adequate for packaging the vast majority of solid drugs and many liquid drugs as well.

2. Some plastics are susceptible to stress cracking in the presence of alcohols, organic acids, ethers and many oils. This is a minor problem which can be overcome at no additional cost by choosing the right plastic. Polypropylene, for example, is a low cost versatile packaging plastic that is not subject to environmental stress cracking.

3. No plastic can match glass for immunity to heat, sunlight, and oxygen. Plastics makers use additives that improve the resistance of their products to environmental breakdown but additives can be leached from plastics by certain solvents used in drug formulations.

4. As extremely poor conductors of electricity, plastics tenaciously retain electrostatic charges that attract undesirable dust particles. This tendency can be diminished by incorporating antistatic additives during manufacture, but these additives can lead to interaction problems similar to those noted above.

5. In addition to additives which can be leached out by some solvents, plastics also contain traces of low molecular weight polymer fragments that are more soluble in drug solvents than are the very high molecular weight polymers that constitute most of the plastic. In most cases, this problem can be minimized during the polymer manufacturing process to produce a "pharmaceutical grade" product. Since this requires extra care and cost, there is always the hazard that some manufacturers may cut corners or that the wrong grade

may inadvertently be shipped to a drug packager. Not only does this require constant vigilance by drug companies, it also concerns FDA officials who regard proposed plastic drug packages with particularly intense scrutiny. This in turn requires more effort by drug companies to qualify a plastic package.

The cautious attitude of the FDA and drug manufacturers towards plastic containers for liquid products does not arise solely from the possibility that a plastics manufacturer may be cutting corners or making mistakes, but it is one factor in that attitude and is reflected in the more voluminous procedures established by the FDA to regulate plastic drug container materials.

In the packaging world broadly, paper is used more often than any other material, but except for labels, paper plays an insignificant role in *primary* drug packaging. Were plastics unknown, paper would be used to some degree as a flexible packaging material for drugs, but the superior moisture resistance and moisture permeation barrier of plastic films enable them not only to dominate these applications but also to establish flexible packaging as an important alternative for pharmaceutical packages. For example, the blister package would not exist if paper and aluminum foil were the only flexible packaging materials available.

Paper, of course, is still the best for secondary and tertiary drug packages: the carton that contains the primary package and the corrugated shipping container that contains both.

Plastic Materials—Their Nature and Manufacture

This section will cover plastic resins, films, and composites, the three principal starting materials for plastic container manufacture. The next chapter will cover the making of containers from these materials and from glass and metal.

Plastic Resins—General

Plastic resins consist of polymer molecules formed by joining small molecules (monomers) end to end to form a long chain. For polyethylene, the minimum useful chain length is 1000 monomer units. The molecular weight of commercially useful polymers is in the range of 10,000 to one million. The principal determinants of polymer properties are the molecular weight, the nature of the monomers used to make the polymer, and the polymer manufacturing process. Polymers used in drug packaging are usually made from a single monomer, but copolymers containing more than one monomer are common in other plastics applications.

Polyethylene (PE)

Polyethylene (PE) dominates drug packaging because it offers the essential properties required by most drugs at the lowest cost. PE consists of a long chain of repeating CH_2 units:

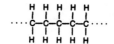

FIGURE 4.1. Polyethylene.

and is made by the polymerization of ethylene:

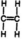

FIGURE 4.2. Ethylene.

If ethylene is polymerized at high pressures and temperatures around 300°F in the presence of a free radical promoter, a polymer containing many branches and side chains is formed, leading to less efficient molecular packing and a low density (0.91–0.93) in the solid resin. This plastic is called *low density polyethylene* (LDPE). Its low cost and good combination of properties make it the world's most frequently used plastic.

If ethylene is polymerized at lower pressures and temperatures in a solvent with a coordination catalyst rather than a free radical catalyst, a polymer molecule with fewer branches and side chains is formed, leading to a higher density resin. This resin is called *high density polyethylene* (HDPE) and is the most widely used plastic resin in drug packaging.

Of these two forms of PE, LDPE is softer, more flexible, more readily stretched and has better clarity. HDPE is stronger, stiffer, less clear, less permeable to gases, more resistant to oils, chemicals, and solvents, can be sterilized by autoclaving and is 5–10%

Table 4.1. Comparison of LDPE and HDPE [3].

Property	LDPE	HDPE
Density, g/cc	0.91–0.925	0.945–0.967
Tensile Strength, kpsi	1.2–2.5	3.0–7.5
Tensile Modulus,		
1% Secant, kpsi	20–40	125
Haze, %	4–10	25–50
WVTR, g-mil/100 in²-day		
@ 100°F & 90% RH	1.2	0.3–0.65

higher in cost (see Table 4.1). Both forms of PE are widely compatible with drugs and are acceptable to the FDA from this standpoint, although stability must be demonstrated in a NDA since PE is somewhat permeable to moisture and oxygen.

The greater strength, stiffness, and moisture barrier of HDPE have led to its widespread use in bottles for solid dosage forms. Although these containers do not have LDPE's clarity, this is not a drawback—in fact, HDPE bottles are usually pigmented or printed white to block light transmission and improve label clarity.

LDPE is usually the plastic of choice for squeeze bottles because of its soft, flexible character and lower cost.

From the drug packaging standpoint, both forms of PE have drawbacks, many of which are related to permeability:

- They have high permeability to free halogens, precluding their use for solutions containing iodine or chlorine.
- They are permeable to chloroform and ether and cannot be used to store chlorodyne.
- They are softened by castor oil and permeable to coconut oil and certain essential oils used in pharmaceuticals for flavoring or for their favorable aromas, such as oil of peppermint.
- They cannot be used to package highly oxygen-sensitive products.
- They have a poor odor barrier, so any product packaged in them and stored near an odoriferous material may be tainted.

Their other drawbacks are related to their tendency to absorb certain essential or deleterious materials:

- They will sorb certain bactericides (phenylmercuric nitrate, benzalkonium chloride, benzyl alcohol, phenylethyl alcohol); small concentrations of steroids and certain alkaloids (pilocarpine, hyoscine, strophanthin, ouabain); and vegetable and other coloring matter from vegetable drug preparations such as tinctures of belladonna, hysocyamus, and opium. This sorption tendency will vary with molecular weight and can be minimized by using HDPE.
- Their resistance to strong oxidizing acids is poor.
- Their tendency to stress crack in the presence of certain solvents must be offset by using more expensive, higher molecular weight, low melt index grades.

Linear Low Density Polyethylene (LLDPE)

When unsaturated comonomers such as butene, hexene, or octene are added to ethylene in the HDPE process at pressures around 300 psi and with altered reaction conditions and catalyst, a third form of PE is produced. Its density is in the same range as LDPE but the degree of side-chain branching is greatly reduced, which accounts for its name. The result is a resin that combines the clarity of LDPE with the toughness of HDPE. LLDPE's use in drug packaging is due to another attribute: it makes very strong heat seals at low temperatures which, like the ionomer heat seals discussed below, have good *hot tack*, the ability of the seal to remain intact as it cools down from its sealing temperature.

Ionomers

When ethylene is polymerized with other unsaturated hydrocarbon comonomers, the family of ethylene copolymers is created. One of these, an ionomer tradenamed Surlyn® [4], is used in drug packaging as a heat seal coating on LDPE and oriented polypropylene (OPP) for pouches and other applications where a strong, hermetic seal with excellent hot tack is important enough to justify the additional cost.

Ionomers are ethylene methacrylic acid (EMAA) copolymers that have some of the hydrogen atoms on the carboxyl groups replaced by either sodium or zinc atoms. This can be done either by adding a sodium or zinc compound to the high pressure polymerization reactor along with ethylene and the appropriate acid comonomer or by partially neutralizing the acid copolymer with a sodium or zinc compound in a second step after the copolymer is made. The result is the structure shown in Figure 4.3.

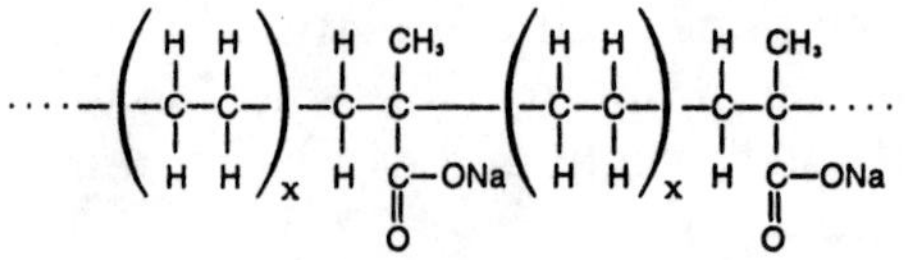

FIGURE 4.3. Ionomer structure.

The high cost of this specialized material (about three times that of LDPE) limits its use to those drug packaging applications that demand excellent seal integrity or greatly enhanced puncture resistance.

Polyvinyl Chloride

This plastic, universally called *vinyl* and abbreviated PVC is, next to HDPE, the most frequently used plastic for drug packaging, consuming about 30 million lbs of resin annually, two-thirds of which is used in rigid packages and one-third in flexible packages, the latter being largely IV bags [5]. This is about 10% of the total annual PVC film and sheet production but less than 1% of the total PVC production in the U.S.

The reasons for PVC's widespread use in drug packaging are clarity, low cost, great fabrication flexibility and tradition. The latter is the reason OPP has not penetrated the flexible vinyl market which is vulnerable because of the vinyl chloride monomer problem discussed below.

Manufacture and Properties

PVC is made at moderate pressures by the free radical polymerization of a vinyl chloride (Figure 4.4) emulsion in water at 60°C:

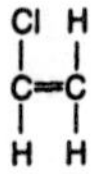

FIGURE 4.4. Structure of vinyl chloride.

to form the long chain polymer shown in Figure 4.5:

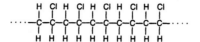

FIGURE 4.5. Structure of PVC.

Unplasticized PVC is a very clear, stiff material with a low water vapor transmission rate (WVTR), comparable to LDPE but is denser by about 30% than PE because of its chlorine content. These properties of unplasticized PVC, along with its excellent thermoformability; high flexural strength; good chemical resistance; low permeability to oils, fats, and flavoring ingredients; easy tintability and low cost make it the material of choice for blister packaging, where it has essentially 100% of the market for the plastic component. For this application it can be readily combined with high barrier plastics such as polyvinylidene chloride (PVDC) and ACLAR® [6,13] to provide a package with ample resistance to penetration by both oxygen and water vapor.

Possible competitors for the blister application are polyethylene terephthalate (PET) and polypropylene (PP). These are now in test here and in Europe but used very little as yet. Two different blister packages for lozenge products now incorporate PP as a substitute for PVC.

PVC is used in clear bottles rather than PET or HDPE when the packager needs better clarity than HDPE offers and wants to avoid the expense of the costly orientation process that PET requires. For opaque bottles, PVC (vs. HDPE) provides a better odor barrier, absorbs fewer flavor components and makes a glossier bottle for better store shelf appearance. HDPE, on the other hand, can be autoclave sterilized, does not require PVC's extensive array of additives and is moderately lower in cost.

For use as a flexible film in IV solution bags, PVC is plasticized with dioctyl phthalate, dioctyl adipate or di-2-ethylhexyl phthalate at levels up to 50%. Levels of plasticizer this high markedly increase PVC's permeability to water vapor and make users generally nervous about the possibility of these low molecular weight materials leaching into the bag contents. For this reason, one producer has adopted a plasticizer based on a citric acid ester for blood bags, but is not switching plasticizers in its IV bags because it claims that no migration occurs with nonfatty fluids such as saline or glucose solutions [7].

For processing into film or sheet, PVC must be heat stabilized, usually with organotin compounds, and must also contain lubricants. On top of all this, traces of vinyl chloride monomer (VCM) are always present. This compound is a human carcinogen, so VCM levels are now always kept below 50 ppb and usually below 10 ppb. The 50 ppb level is not specifically regulated but nevertheless is carefully adhered to by all PVC manufacturers [8].

The major drug packaging application for rigid PVC with low plasticizer content is in blister packaging. Flexible PVC with high plasticizer content is used mostly in IV solution bags. PVC dominates these two applications in spite of its high additive level and the VCM problem. For blisters, it has excellent thermoformability and coatability. For IV bags, it has a good combination of mechanical properties and it is entrenched. Polypropylene is beginning to appear as a competitive material for bags. When its FDA approval process has been completed, the bag market will gradually shift to PP because of the plasticizer/additive issue in PVC [9]. In the blister application, on the other hand, PVC's position as the dominant plastic is so far unchallenged.

Polypropylene (PP)

This plastic is widely used as film for food packaging and many other industrial uses. It is used in drug packaging for closures and box overwrap, tablet vials, and for IV solution bottles where the breakability of glass is a major drawback.

Manufacture and Properties

Although similar to PE, PP has a more complex structure. When propylene molecules shown in Figure 4.6 combine to form PP at about 200 psi in a hydrocarbon solvent in the presence of a coordination catalyst, the CH_3 side groups follow a regular pattern.

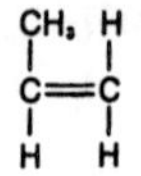

$$
\begin{array}{cc}
CH_3 & H \\
| & | \\
C\!\!=\!\!C \\
| & | \\
H & H
\end{array}
$$

FIGURE 4.6. The propylene molecule.

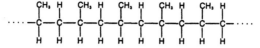

FIGURE 4.7. The structure of PP.

The PP molecules (Figure 4.7), especially after orientation, are packed regularly in an ordered crystalline structure producing strong, stiff, clear films. In both film and container form, this plastic is clearer than HDPE and stronger, tougher, stiffer and more high temperature-resistant than LDPE. It has a gas barrier similar to HDPE and superior to that of LDPE. Its stiffness and clarity make it an attractive box overwrap film. Its combination of strength, good flex crack resistance and relatively low cost account for its widespread use in closures, particularly for those with hinges which must resist repeated flexing.

Compared to PE, PP has:

- better resistance to greases and oils
- comparable resistance to solvents
- poorer resistance to oxidation and oxidizing reagents
- better odor barrier
- less tendency to absorb active ingredients of aqueous bactericide solutions (chlorhexidene acetate, methyl paraben, phenyl mercuric nitrate, benzalkonium chloride, etc.)
- better resistance to elevated temperatures by about 30°F
- lower additive content

When used as a film, PP is usually oriented to enhance its mechanical properties. In that form (OPP), it has one drawback: it is difficult to heat seal. This problem can be avoided by using PP/PE copolymers that have a broad heat seal range, lower melting point, lower modulus and better impact strength. These can either be coextruded with PP or applied separately as coatings.

The largest *potential* market for OPP film in drug packaging is as a replacement for flexible PVC. This is a likely eventuality, encouraged by packagers concerned about vinyl chloride monomer and desirous of a material with additive content.

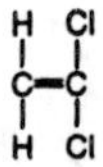

$$
\begin{array}{c}
\text{H} \quad \text{Cl} \\
| \quad | \\
\text{C}\!-\!\text{C} \\
| \quad | \\
\text{H} \quad \text{Cl}
\end{array}
$$

FIGURE 4.8. The vinylidene chloride molecule.

Polyvinylidene Chloride (PVDC)

Although the volume of this specialized plastic in drug packaging is small, it plays a critical role in blister and strip packaging as laminations or coatings on PVC or OPP to improve gas barrier. It is also widely used for gas barrier in wad facings. In these applications, PVDC is used as a copolymer with PVC, which it closely resembles in monomer form, as shown in Figure 4.8.

Compared to most plastics, PVDC, like PVC, has a high density (1.7 g/cc) and is expensive on an area basis. For these reasons, it is rarely used as a film by itself or as a drug container since HDPE, LDPE, PP and PVC can all provide an adequate moisture barrier at lower cost and oxygen barrier is rarely important in drug packages.

Polystyrene (PS)

Polystyrene was one of the earliest plastics to be commercialized. It is made by the peroxide-catalyzed polymerization of styrene (Figure 4.9).

PS is an amorphous, crystal clear, hard, brittle, stiff material with low impact resistance, easy thermoformability, and, compared to HDPE, only one-tenth the moisture barrier and one-third the oxygen barrier. It is used in drug packaging, often tinted amber, for tubes and bottles where clarity and stiffness are important and poor gas barrier is no drawback. It is also used for jars for ointments and creams with low water content and no organic sol-

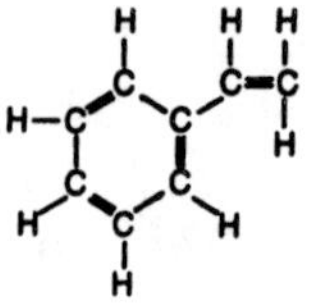

FIGURE 4.9. The styrene molecule.

vents. Although it is still used for packaging medical devices because of its clarity, thermoformability, and low cost (about half that of PVC), its use in drug packaging is limited and declining because of its poor gas barrier, poor solvent resistance and low softening point, which precludes heat sterilization.

Polyesters

These polymers are made by reacting a diacid or diester with a bifunctional alcohol and then polymerizing the resultant monomer. The most common and lowest cost polyester is made by reacting dimethyl terephthalate (DMT):

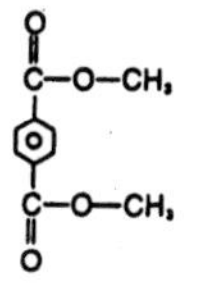

FIGURE 4.10. The DMT molecule.

with ethylene glycol:

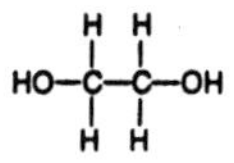

FIGURE 4.11. Ethylene glycol.

to eliminate methanol and form polyethylene terephthalate (PET):

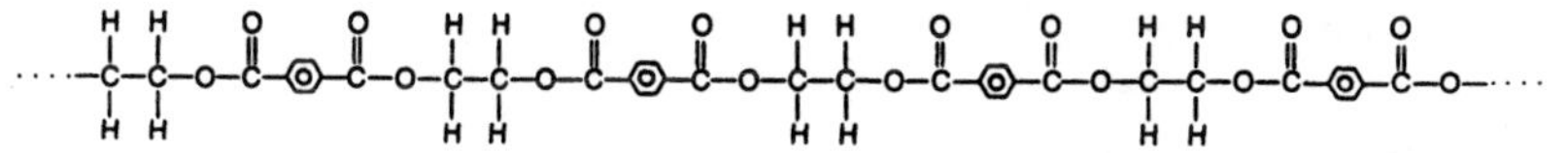

FIGURE 4.12. The structure of PET.

This plastic is used in a wide variety of industrial, electronic, and food packaging applications, notably as the popular plastic soft drink bottle where its strength, clarity and good CO_2 barrier make it the best choice among the various plastic candidates.

Oriented PET forms a strong, clear, tough film with good moisture barrier that retains its mechanical properties at relatively high temperatures. As a container, it develops the same mechanical properties only if the container is oriented during manufacture. This is a relatively expensive process, so alternatives such as PVC, PP, HDPE or LDPE will usually be used if they are functional. However, as container sizes continue to be standardized and volume continues to increase, PET will become more popular in preference to PVC when good clarity is essential. One reason for this is the perception that PET is more recyclable than PVC. A good example is the choice of PET for Plax, an anti-plaque dental rinse, to replace PVC for this product in the U.K. Currently, Germany and the U.S. use PET for Plax, even at a cost penalty, because PET is more readily recycled in those countries [10].

The excellent CO_2 barrier of PET which is vital for carbonated beverages is irrelevant in drug packaging. PET's good high temperature properties are frequently important for food but rarely for drugs. Thus PET will always be far more widely used for food than for drugs.

Related to PET is PETG, a copolymer of PET and cyclohexane dimethanol. Amorphous in nature as opposed to PET, this polymer yields film and sheet which are very clear, tough, impact resistant, stable to irradiation sterilization, readily thermoformable, lower in cost than polycarbonate, and which contain no stabilizers or fillers. It could also be a candidate to replace PVC in applications where plasticizer migration is of concern [11]. Although its water vapor transmission rate (WVTR) of 4 g-mil/100 in²-24 hr is comparable to PVC, it is ten times higher than HDPE and four times higher than PET. Thus, like PVC, PETG must be coated if WVTR is crucial. PETG is currently about 20% more expensive than PVC on a coverage basis.

Polyamides

Commonly known by the generic name *nylon*, most polyamides are made by reacting two different monomers, an acid and an amine, to eliminate water. For the most common nylon, the two monomers are hexamethylenediamine:

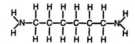

FIGURE 4.13. Hexamethylenediamine.

and adipic acid:

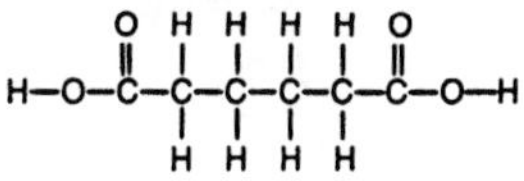

FIGURE 4.14. Adipic acid.

These are reacted together and then polymerized to form the long chain 6,6 nylon:

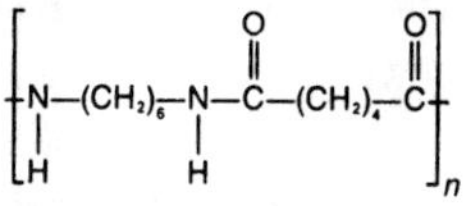

FIGURE 4.15. 6,6 nylon.

Like polyesters, polyamides find widespread use as engineering plastics but are infrequently used in drug packaging because of their very poor moisture barrier and relatively high cost. Drug packaging rarely demands the good mechanical properties that make polyamides popular and cost-effective in engineering applications.

Fluorine-Containing Polymers

These high-cost specialized materials are widely used in demanding nonpackaging applications where, for example, the low coefficient of friction and outstanding chemical resistance of PTFE (Teflon [12]) lead to its frequent use in corrosive environments and rotating machinery.

In drug packaging, Teflon is used as a liner for rubber stoppers where its inertness to all chemicals and solvents protects the package contents against adulteration by stopper components.

Teflon is made by the polymerization of tetrafluoroethylene:

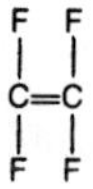

FIGURE 4.16. Tetrafluoroethylene.

The properties of this basic fluorocarbon can be modified by incorporating comonomers such as perfluorinated propylene.

Also of interest in drug packaging is the polymer made from trichlorofluoroethylene:

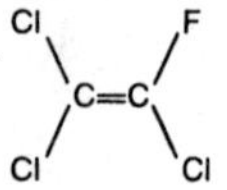

FIGURE 4.17. Trichlorofluoroethylene.

and called ACLAR [13] by its sole U.S. manufacturer. ACLAR has an excellent barrier to water vapor, about equal to that of PVDC. Its oxygen barrier is twice that of PET or 6,6 nylon but only one-tenth that of PVDC. It is inert to most chemicals and has excellent resistance to ozone and ultraviolet light, good transparency and a service temperature up to 300°F.

ACLAR films are difficult to extrude but have good tear strength and moderately good mechanical properties. About one million pounds per year are used in drug packaging as a laminate with PVC in blister packages. In this role the film is an alternative to PVDC in providing the high moisture barrier needed by some products. When laminated to PVC, ACLAR film can provide a moisture barrier about 15–20% better than the thickest practical PVDC coatings at only a modest increase in cost. Thus packagers frequently use ACLAR when introducing a sensitive new drug or when they feel they must have the best barrier possible regardless of cost [14].

Low sales volume and high intermediate costs put the price of ACLAR so high that it is never used by itself for containers requiring high barrier properties.

Polyurethane

Polyurethane is another example, like ACLAR, of a plastic with a very specialized but important application in drug packaging. Polyurethanes are made by reacting diisocyanates:

$$O=C=N-R-N=C=O$$

FIGURE 4.18. A diisocyanate.

with glycols:

$$HO-CH_2-CH_2-OH$$

FIGURE 4.19. A glycol.

to form the polymer:

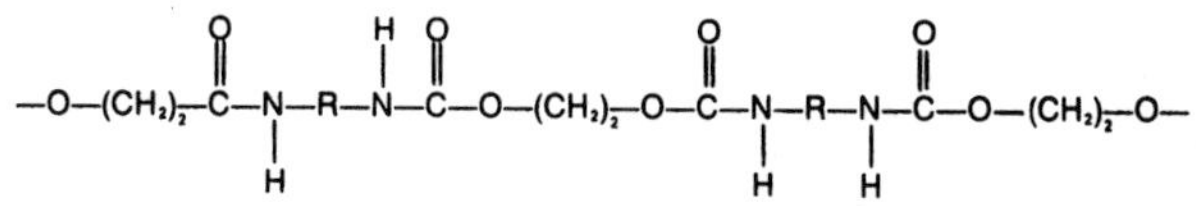

FIGURE 4.20. A polyurethane.

Many isocyanates and glycols are available to make polyurethanes with a variety of properties.

Under certain conditions and with certain reactants, the polymerization reaction evolves CO_2 and produces a foam. Foamed polyurethane can be a flexible, open-cell material or a rigid, closed-cell material. Flexible polyurethane foam, along with fibers of rayon, polyester, and polyurethane, are now used in preference to cotton for tablet bottle stuffing because they do not absorb moisture the way cotton does. The only problem with polyurethanes is light sensitivity, so these foam stuffings are either used in opaque bottles or supplied tinted to mask light-catalyzed discoloration [15].

The right choice of polyurethane monomers produces films that have a very high permeability to the active components of drugs designed for transdermal delivery.

THE MANUFACTURE OF
PLASTIC FILMS

Overview

This section is not a manual of film manufacture. It is intended to provide an overview of this subject to give the reader some understanding of the processes involved. Detailed descriptions are available in modern works on the subject [16].

Three categories of flexible substrates are used in drug packaging: plastic films, paper, and aluminum foil. Of these three, plastics play a dominant role. In 1989, plastic films held 86% of the $430 million market for flexible substrates in drug packaging, aluminum foil held 13%, and paper only 1% [17]. The $370 million share held by plastics is broken down as follows [18]:

- LDPE and HDPE: 46%
- PVC: 8%
- PET: 9.5%
- PS: 9.5%
- PP: 7%
- all others: 20%

Film Manufacture

The most common way of making plastic films is to extrude the molten plastic through a die that creates a relatively thick, 1–5 mil, film which is subsequently reduced to the final desired thickness by stretching the film while it is still molten in the direction of its travel and often also in the direction transverse to travel. The film at final thickness is then wound up on rolls and later slit to the desired width.

Mixing and extrusion of the plastic resins and other essential ingredients take place in an extruder, which consists of a metal screw rotating inside a metal cylinder, as shown in Figure 4.21.

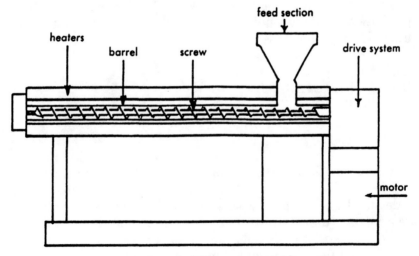

FIGURE 4.21. A typical film extruder (schematic).

After the ingredients are thoroughly mixed, the extruder forces the molten mixture through a die, which can either be flat or circular [see Figures 4.22(a) and 4.22(b)], melt drawn, quenched and wound up (Figures 4.23 and 4.24).

Flat dies are used when very close tolerances are required, but their complexity leads producers to use, where possible, circular dies that form a tube of plastic rather than a sheet. This tube is called a *bubble*.

Some plastic films, such as PET and PP, can have their mechanical properties enhanced by a process known as orientation. This is a state in which the polymer molecules in the film are aligned. It is brought about by heating the cool, as-cast film, stretching it in both machine and transverse directions while it is warm, and then holding it in biaxial tension while it is heat-set at a higher temperature. In the flat die process, orientation requires a complex piece of equipment called a *tenter frame*. In the circular die process, the rewarmed film in tubular form can be stretched in both directions by a combination of downstream pulling with rollers and air pressure inside the tube which expands it in the transverse direction. Equipment to accomplish this two-way stretch, while not simple, is easier to operate and maintain than the tenter frame.

Certain films can be oriented so that when heated, they shrink to 60–80% of their original dimensions. When wrapped around an object to be packaged, sealed, and heated in a shrink tunnel, these films shrink around the object and faithfully adapt to its contours. PVC, PP, LDPE and LDPE/HDPE blends are all used to make shrink films.

PVC film and sheet are also made, not by the extrusion of a melt through a die, but by a process known as *calendering*. Here the ingredients are blended in the molten state in batch equipment. Large blobs of the molten blend are then fed to a series of rolls which form the sheet by spreading the blob and extending it longitudinally as in the extruder process described above.

The calender is a complex machine involving as many as 30 separate rolls. The main rolls operate at high temperatures and must be constantly adjusted to be sure the correct film thickness is produced. Following these main rolls is a complex set of take-off rolls, tempering rolls, and cooling rolls, all with different diameters and all running at different temperatures and speeds. The end result is a film or sheet of precisely controlled thickness and properties designed for a specific end use [20]. Although the

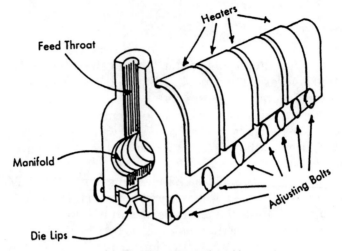

(a) Flat die cross-sectioned in
middle at feed throat

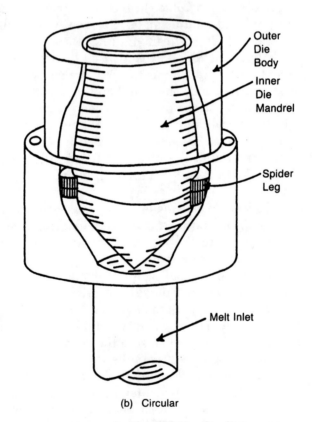

(b) Circular

FIGURE 4.22. Flat and circular dies.

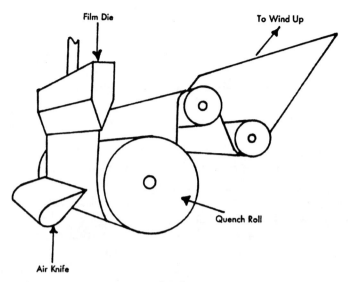

FIGURE 4.23. The flat die process.

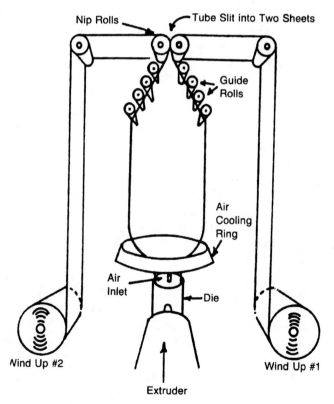

FIGURE 4.24. The circular die process.

quality of calendered sheet and film is superior to that produced by extrusion, the process is more expensive to operate and the complex equipment is more expensive to maintain.

Additives and Modifiers

Most plastic films must have materials added to them, usually in the extrusion step, to improve their properties, to facilitate the film-forming process, and to modify surface characteristics.

Lubricants assist in the molding and extrusion steps. Examples are stearic acids and their derivatives.

Slip agents, usually silica, reduce the coefficient of friction of the plastic and reduce its tendency to stick to itself.

Antistatic agents such as quaternary ammonium compounds reduce the buildup of static charges on the surface of the plastic film.

Surface treatments, such as exposure to a corona discharge or application of very thin layers of other plastics, improve the ink receptivity of the film, its adherence to other films, its heat sealability or its gas barrier properties.

Stabilizers increase the resistance of the plastic to degradation by heat or light. These can be epoxidized soybean oil, organotin compounds or benzoates of barium or cadmium.

Plasticizers enhance flexibility, resiliency and melt flow. The most common plasticizers are high boiling organic liquids, usually phthalates, of which dioctyl phthalate is the most popular.

Antioxidants, which are easily oxidized materials such as aromatic amines, hindered phenolics, thioesters or phosphites, retard the oxidation of plastics by inhibiting the formation of free radicals that cause oxidative breakdown.

Dyes and pigments impart color or opacity to these normally clear, colorless materials.

All these additives are of concern in drug packaging because of their potential for migrating into the drug and altering its potency, stability or efficacy. This concern is greater for liquid preparations and is particularly acute for parenteral liquids. Polystyrene and PVC contain more additives than do polyolefins or PET. The complex FDA testing and approval procedures discussed in Chapter Three help assure that these additives will not contaminate the package contents.

Composite Films

One reason for the popularity of flexible packaging is the development of composite films: combinations of different plastic films that may include paper and/or aluminum foil. Use of a composite film often makes it easier to attain all the properties required of a packaging film: strength, stiffness, heat sealability, gas barrier, controlled light transmission and low cost. In drug packaging, the principal function of composite films is to increase gas barrier in blister packages and flexible tubes.

Manufacture of Composite Films

Composite film structures are made by three basic methods: coating, lamination, and coextrusion.

Coating

Coatings applied to plastic films are usually other polymers that increase gas barrier and enhance heat sealability. In drug packaging, PVDC is the most common coating because it performs both these functions very well.

PVDC coatings can reduce the moisture permeability (WVTR) of PVC blister packages manyfold, as shown in Table 4.2 [21]. In this table and in the rest of this book, multilayer plastic structures are described by identifying each layer, starting from the outside and working in, and separating the layers with the "/". Thus PVC adhesively laminated on the outside with PVDC would be written PVDC/adh/PVC.

Table 4.2. WVTR of PVC composites.

Material	WVTR[1]
PVC	0.2–0.3
PVDC/adh/PVC[2]	0.03–0.04 (PVDC @ 40–60 g/m²)
PVDC/adh/PE/adh/PVC[2,3]	0.006–0.03 (PVDC @ 40–90 g/m²)

[1]The units of WVTR are g-mil/100 in²–24 hr measured at 90% RH and 38°C.
[2]In the two PVDC-coated cases, the numbers in parentheses are the PVDC coating thickness expressed as grams per square meter.
[3]In the third structure, PE absorbs the shock of flexing that would crack the relatively brittle PVDC layer.

Coatings are applied to films either as water emulsions, as solutions in organic solvents, as molten materials (extrusion coating) or from the vapor phase by deposition in a vacuum chamber. Selection of the process to be used depends on the characteristics of the substrate, the properties of the coating material and the equipment available to the coater.

In the first two methods, the substrate film is unwound and run through a bath containing the coating material, then through rolls which adjust the coating thickness and ensure its uniformity, and then through a drying tower which evaporates the solvent or water. Alternatively, the coating can be applied by gravure rolls which rotate in the coating bath.

In extrusion coating, the molten coating material is extruded through a die and falls on the substrate as it passes below the die. A series of downstream rolls then cool the coated substrate and adjust coating thickness.

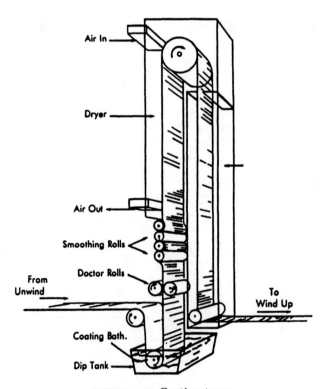

FIGURE 4.25. Coating tower.

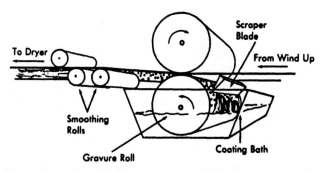

FIGURE 4.26. Gravure coating.

Figures 4.25, 4.26, and 4.27 illustrate these processes.

In the examples cited in Table 4.2, the PVDC coatings are applied by dispersion coating, the adhesives by solvent or dispersion coating and the PE by adhesive lamination.

The fourth process is called *metallization* because it is used only to apply submicron coatings of aluminum to plastic or paper substrates. The process takes place in large chambers which can be evacuated to pressures of 0.01 atmospheres or lower. Under these conditions, aluminum atoms vaporize from a molten pool and condense on a film of plastic that is slowly unwound above the molten pool. The thickness of the deposit is controlled by the

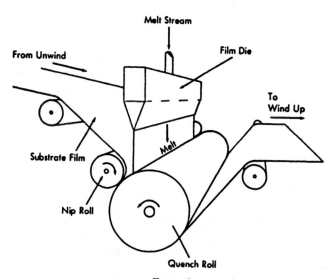

FIGURE 4.27. Extrusion coating.

rate at which fresh film surface is exposed to the vaporizing aluminum.

Since the aluminum layer can be made very thin and can be created without the expensive foil manufacturing process, metallized films cost substantially less than foil. The moisture and oxygen barriers that can be achieved with metallized coatings are more than sufficient for most drug packaging applications. However, metallization has not been adopted by drug packagers because of their general conservatism and the lengthy testing and FDA approval process that would be required.

Lamination

Lamination is the joining together, with heat and adhesives, of two or more dissimilar flexible substrates. The adhesives can be thermoplastic materials such as vinyl acetate/vinyl chloride copolymers, polyesters or polyurethanes which are applied to the separate materials prior to lamination (adhesive lamination, see Figure 4.28) or can be low melting plastic resins such as PE that are added to the sandwich either in film form or extruded into the space between the layers to be joined together during the lamination process (extrusion lamination, see Figure 4.29).

Lamination is the most versatile of the composite film manufacturing processes because a wide variety of materials, including nonthermoplastic substrates such as paper and foil, can be successfully joined together by the use of adhesives and heat. For example, a common lamination in drug packaging is a combination of paper, plastic and foil used for lidding in thermoformed structures, the backing layer for blisters, and as a sachet pouch. Foil supplies the gas barrier, plastics furnish toughness, adhesive character, and protection for the foil and paper provides stiffness and bulk.

Coextrusion

Although quite versatile, lamination is a relatively expensive process since the individual webs must be made, wound up and then unwound to feed the process. Coextrusion, a newer process, avoids these added costs by creating the composite structure in one step, as shown in Figure 4.30.

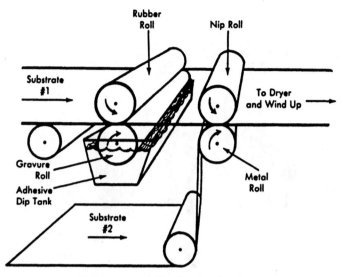

FIGURE 4.28. Adhesive lamination.

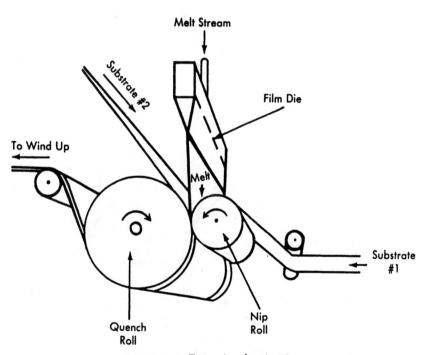

FIGURE 4.29. Extrusion lamination.

131

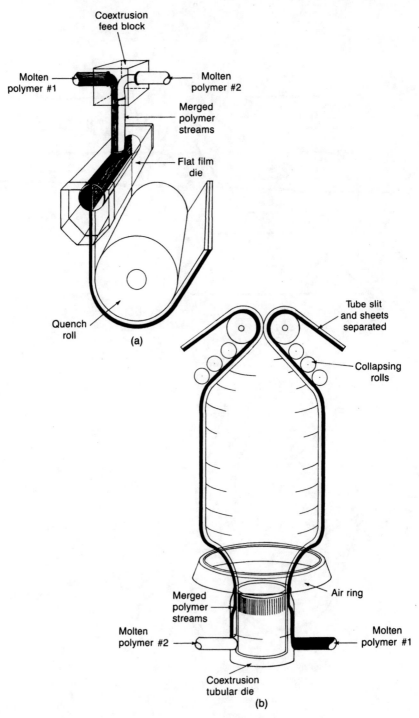

FIGURE 4.30. The coextrusion process: (a) flat die process; (b) tubular process.

132

As shown, several streams of different molten polymers (including polymers which may be needed to provide adhesion between the functional layers which may be quite dissimilar chemically) are simultaneously fed to a complex die where they are joined together to form a multilayer film. Remarkably, the film layers do not intermix during this process but rather form a tightly bonded, layered structure which closely resembles a lamination. Coextrusions are lower in cost since the prior manufacture of the separate components in film form is avoided. The absence of solvents used in adhesive lamination is also a plus, since control of solvent emissions from converter plants is now closely regulated by the EPA.

Coextrusion has a few disadvantages which preclude its totally displacing lamination:

- Not all components of the desired composite may be extrudable. Paper, foil, and cellulosic films are the most obvious examples. Even some important thermoplastic resins such as PVDC must be modified, with some loss in barrier properties, to make them extrudable.
- Not all extrudable thermoplastic resins will adhere tightly to one another in this process. This drawback is rapidly disappearing as the family of coextrudable adhesives expands to cover all cases of commercial interest.
- Coextruded films must be printed after they are made, which means that the printing is always on the surface of the film where it is subject to abrasion in handling. In a lamination, one layer can be printed prior to lamination and the printed surface can then be sandwiched between the other layers to protect it from abrasion.
- If one of the plastic film components must be oriented to develop desired properties, this may be more complicated if other plastic layers are already present.

The use of coextrusions in drug packaging lies mainly in the future, which will also bring a gradual shift of rigid to flexible packaging and lead to more frequent use of multilayer structures, both laminated and coextruded.

The Permeability of Plastics

Throughout this chapter, repeated reference has been made to the permeation rate of plastic films to oxygen and water vapor. The natural permeability of plastics, compared to impervious glass and metal, make permeability an important consideration when choosing a plastic packaging material.

For a small molecule such as water or oxygen to permeate a plastic film, it must be soluble in the film and be able to diffuse through it. Aggregates of polymer chains that are flexible will readily open up to allow diffusion of these small molecules through the structure, but stiff, bulky chains are less accommodating. Thus the barrier of any polymer to permeation by gases can be enhanced by increasing the degree of crystallinity of the polymer structure or by adding bulky groups to the backbone of the chain that will interfere with chain movement. In practice it is often less expensive to coat the base film with another polymer that has these characteristics to produce a multilayer structure with enhanced barrier to gas permeation.

The testing process for moisture permeability of rigid containers is described in Chapters Three and Eight. The moisture permeability of sheets or films can be measured by sealing the film sample over the mouth of a metal cup which contains a desiccant. The test cell so formed is then treated just like the container in the USP test.

One common test for oxygen permeability involves separating two chambers by a sample of the film to be tested and establishing a known partial pressure of oxygen on one side of the film and zero partial pressure of oxygen on the other. Then, as oxygen diffuses through the film in response to the pressure gradient so established, a detector on the zero side that is sensitive to oxygen (or any other gas, such as CO_2, that may be of interest) continuously records the buildup of the permeant gas.

Water vapor transmission rates (WVTR) are commonly reported in units of g-mil/100 in^2–24 hr to normalize the measurement to a film of 1 mil thickness and a specific area (100 in^2) over a specific time period (24 hr). Grams represent the amount of water picked up by the desiccant. Oxygen or other gas permeability rates are expressed in units of cc-mil/100 in^2–24 hr-atm. Temperature and relative humidity, both of which affect the rate, must be specified.

ELASTOMERIC MATERIALS

Overview

The material in this section has been derived largely from an excellent review article by Smith [23], to which the reader is referred for additional detail. Elastomers are polymers that can be stretched to at least twice their unstretched length and return to their original length when the stretching force is released. This high stretchability differentiates elastomers from other materials used in drug packaging; metal and plastics are elastic only over a very small deformation range.

In drug packaging, elastomers are used mainly for parenteral container closures. This use arises from two unique physical properties of elastomers—compressability and resealability. Their compressability allows them to seal small irregularities in mating surfaces such as the inside of the neck of a parenteral vial. Reclosability allows them to close completely after a hypodermic needle has been withdrawn.

General Description of Elastomers

Elastomers are complex materials containing from two to ten different raw materials. They are classified as saturated or unsaturated depending on the frequency of the double bond content in the polymer chain. The degree of unsaturation determines both their physical and their chemical properties. Highly unsaturated elastomers have "rubbery" mechanical properties but poor resistance to water, solvents, and oils. Examples of the two types are shown in Table 4.3 [24].

A detailed listing of the properties of these and more elastomers can be found in Reference [25]. Properties of importance for pharmaceutical applications are:

- impermeability to gases
- coring resistance (resistance to fragmentation when penetrated by a needle)
- compression recovery

Table 4.3. Saturated and unsaturated elastomers.

Saturated	Unsaturated
Butyl	Natural
Halogenated Butyls	Styrene-Butadiene
Ethylene-Propylene Rubber	Polyisoprene
Silicone	Neoprene

- shelf life
- solvent resistance
- resilience
- resistance to ozone and radiation
- resistance to interaction with the package contents

The last property can be improved by coating the closure with cured epoxy resins or Teflon to interpose a barrier between the closure and the package contents.

**The Chemical Structure
of Elastomers**

Some typical elastomeric chemical structures are shown in Table 4.4 [26].

Of these various types of elastomers, butyl and chlorobutyl rubbers share 80% of the overall parenteral closure market since they offer the best resistance to permeation by oxygen and water vapor. When multiple penetration by a needle is required, natural rubber is included in the chlorobutyl formulation to give better coring resistance. If the drug contains mineral oil, then nitrile rubber or neoprene is used.

For large IV fluid containers that require a 28 or 32 mm stopper, EPDM rubber is the material of choice because it uses a peroxide curing system that minimizes the occurrence of curing compound components that could react with the package contents. Silicone-based elastomers are used largely for contact lens vials because their good heat resistance allows multiple autoclaving for resterilization after the lens has been removed and then replaced. However, the high gas permeability of these materials precludes their use in other pharmaceutical closure applications.

Manufacture of Elastomers

Ingredients and Their Functions

Generally, elastomers can be classified as natural or synthetic. Natural elastomers contain natural rubber, extracted from rubber trees, as the elastomeric component. Synthetic elastomers are produced, like plastics, from petrochemicals. The final product, ready for use as a closure, is made by combining the elastomer with other materials:

Table 4.4. Some typical elastomeric structures.

Elastomer	Structure
Butyl Rubber	$[-(CH_2-C)_{50}-(CH_2-C=CH-CH_2)-]_n$ with CH_3 groups on the C (top and bottom) and CH_3 on the $C=CH$
Halobutyl Rubber	$[-CH_2-C)_{65}-(CH-C-CH-CH_2)-]_n$ with CH_3, CH_3, X, CH_2; $X = Cl$ or Br
Ethylene-Propylene Rubber	$[(CH_2-CH_2)_3(CH_2-CH)]_n$ with CH_3
Silicone Rubber	$[-Si-O-]_n$ with CH_3 (top and bottom)
Fluoroelastomers	$[-C-C-]_n$ with F, F (top) and F, F (bottom)
Natural Rubber	$[-CH_2-C=CH-CH_2-]_n$ with CH_3
Neoprene Rubber	$[-CH_2-C=CH-CH_2-]_n$ with Cl
Styrene Butadiene Rubber	$[(CH_2-CH=CH-CH_2)_4(CH_2-CH)]_n$ with C_6H_5
Polybutadiene	$[-CH_2-CH=CH-CH_2-]_n$

- curing or vulcanizing agents (sulfur, peroxides) which cross-link the elastomer chains under heat
- cure accelerators (amines, thiazoles) and activators (zinc oxide, stearic acid) which speed up the curing process
- antioxidants (hindered phenols, amines) for unsaturated elastomers which preferentially oxidize in place of the elastomer and prolong its shelf life
- plasticizers/lubricants (oils, phthalates) which facilitate mixing and molding of the ingredients
- fillers (carbon black, silicates) which increase hardness and abrasion resistance, improve physical properties and reduce cost
- pigments (TiO_2, inorganic oxides, carbon black) which color the rubber for aesthetic or functional purposes

The choice of these ingredients depends on the elastomer and what its use will be. Typical use factors that must be considered in making ingredient choices are:

- the nature of the drug being packaged
- solvents or preservatives that are present and may react with the elastomer
- the pH of the package contents and the buffer system, if any, that is used to control the pH
- the sensitivity of the package contents to metals
- the degree of protection needed against oxygen and water vapor
- the closure configuration and color

Both the choice of raw materials and manufacturing method used are influenced by FDA regulations just as with other packaging materials. However, there are no FDA regulations concerning elastomers that apply solely to drug packaging; the same regulations apply to food as well. Applicable sections of the CFRs are 21 CFR 175, 177, 178, 182, 184, and 185.

Manufacturing

The manufacture of an elastomeric article, such as a stopper, begins with the mixing of the ingredients in a roll mill or an internal mixer. The mix is then extruded as a sheet which is placed on a multicavity mold where heat and pressure create the desired shape and cure the article. Alternatively, gamma or electron beam radiation can be used to effect curing and cross linking in this step.

Curing cross links the elastomer chains to form a three-dimensional network with the desired physical and chemical properties. The character of the mass changes from plastic to elastomeric. It goes from a tacky, plastic, soluble, inelastic, readily weatherable material to an elastic, slippery, solvent-resistant, weather-resistant product. The physical properties that develop depend on the number and types of cross links; strength and stiffness, for example, increase in proportion to the degree of cross linking.

In the third step, the molded, cured shapes are trimmed from the sheet and washed. Finishing operations are then performed — often stoppers are glazed by chlorination or siliconized to reduce their coefficient of friction and facilitate their handling on high speed filling lines. Some compositions require extraction of objectionable residual materials by autoclaving. Lacquers or Teflon coatings may be applied to prevent interaction with the package contents.

Throughout the manufacturing process, stringent testing and controls are applied to the ingredients, in-process material, and finished product.

Although the unique mechanical properties of elastomers make their use indispensable for certain types of closures, elastomers are not totally inert to liquid drugs. Like plastics, they interact with pharmaceutical formulations in three ways:

- adsorption or absorption of essential components
- permeation of components through the closure and into the environment
- leaching of elastomer components into the drug formulation

The final drawback of elastomers is their finite permeability to water vapor and gases such as oxygen. Unlike plastics, barrier coatings or barrier layers are not a facile solution to this problem, since once penetrated, barrier plastics will generally not reseal themselves as elastomers can. As a practical matter, however, stoppers are usually thick enough to provide an adequate gas barrier even though their inherent gas permeability is much higher than coated plastics.

All these negatives can be offset in part by choice of elastomeric composition and manufacturing method, but extensive testing is required to be sure the interactions with a given drug are within tolerable limits and to allow the specification of an expiration date that is specific to the drug, its container, and its closure.

FUTURE TRENDS

The future will bring the development of polymers for packaging that will have enhanced oxygen barrier, greater stiffness and higher strength. The two high-oxygen-barrier polymers now available—ethylene vinyl alcohol (EVOH) and PVDC—both have drawbacks. PVDC decomposes at elevated temperatures and EVOH loses barrier under high humidity conditions. Although the future will bring improvements in these two materials, it is unlikely that an entirely new polymer will be discovered that incorporates the best features of these two without their drawbacks.

Plastics films with inorganic coatings based on silica will be developed. These will have barrier properties significantly better than PVDC and be more amenable to recycling. Coextrusions that can be successfully surface printed will appear, increasing the popularity of this low cost approach to multilayer films.

The major consumer complaint about plastic film packages is the difficulty encountered in opening them. This will change through the development of better sealant resins to create hermetic seals that are much easier to open.

All of these developments will increase the popularity of plastic pouches for pharmaceutical products, since pouches are the ultimate low cost package. They will also have a positive effect on the blister package, particularly on its use for pharmaceutical liquids.

REFERENCES

1. Sacharow, S. 1985. *Pharmaceutical Manufacturing* (September):14.

2. Osborn, K. R. and W. A. Jenkins. 1992. Chapter 3 in *Plastic Films*. Lancaster, PA: Technomic Publishing Co., Inc. (This chapter provides a discussion of the permeation of gases through plastics.)

3. Ibid., see p. 233 for a more extensive comparison of the properties of various plastics.

4. "Surlyn" is a registered trademark of E. I. du Pont de Nemours & Co., Inc.

5. Knud Christiansen of Klockner-Pentaplast, and Edward Hancock of American Mirrex, private communications, 1991.

6. "ACLAR" is Allied-Signal's tradename for polychlorotrifluoroethylene.

7. Anon. 1992. *Modern Plastics* (March):15.

8. Edward Hancock, American Mirrex, private communication, 1991.

9. R. W. Miller. Fina Oil & Chemical Co., private communication, 1991.

10. Covell, R. L. 1991. *Packaging Digest* (May):50.

11. Anon. 1989. *Manufacturing Chemist* (February):37.

12. "Teflon" is a registered trademark of E. I. du Pont de Nemours & Co., Inc.

13. "ACLAR" is a registered trademark of Allied-Signal Co.

14. Harvey L. Weaver, American Mirrex, private communication, 1992.

15. Wang, Y. J. and Y. W. Chien. 1984. *Technical Report No. 5. Sterile Pharmaceutical Packaging: Compatibility and Stability*. Philadelphia, PA: Parenteral Drug Assn., Inc., p. 130.

16. Osborn, K. R. and W. A. Jenkins. 1992. Chapter 2 in *Plastic Films*. Lancaster, PA: Technomic Publishing Co., Inc.

17. Anon. 1990. *Chemical Week* (July 25):26.

18. Larson, M. 1991. *Packaging* (January):30.

19. These energy content figures include the energy required to obtain and transport the raw materials and to convert them to finished products.

20. Knud Christiansen, Klockner-Pentaplast, private communication, 1991.

21. 1988. Abstracted data from "Quality Certified High Performance Rigid Films for Pharmaceutical Manufacturing," Klockner-Pentaplast company brochure.

22. Here the units for WVTR are g-mil/100 in^2–24 hr measured at 90% RH and 38°C.

23. Smith, E. J. and R. J. Nash. 1986. "Elastomeric Closures for Parenterals," reprinted from K. Avis et al., *Pharmaceutical Dosage Forms*. New York, NY: Marcel Dekker, Chapter 5, p. 155.

24. Ibid., p. 165.

25. Ibid., p. 166.

26. Ibid., p. 169.

CHAPTER FIVE

The Fabrication and Filling
of Pharmaceutical
Containers

The first part of this chapter will cover the methods used to manufacture the containers most commonly used for drugs: glass bottles and vials; metal cans, tubes, and aerosol cans; and plastic bottles, vials, blisters, pouches, and tubes. The second part will describe in summary form how these containers are filled and, where necessary, sterilized.

CONTAINER FABRICATION

The Fabrication of Glass Containers

Glass containers are made by either of two methods:

- Inserting a blob of molten glass into a mold and then using air pressure — "blowing" — to force the blob to assume the contours of the mold. This method is used for bottles and jars.
- Starting with a tube of hot glass and shaping the container from it. This method is used for ampules, vials, and cartridge tubes.

The high melting point of Type I glass makes blowing difficult, so Type I containers are usually made by the second process. The more ready fabricability of Types II and III glasses, makes these types popular for bottles and jars.

Glass tubing, the starting point for the tubular process, is made by flowing molten glass past a rotating, hollow, water-cooled mandrel. The finished tubing is cut to stock lengths which can then be cut and heated to shape and seal the final containers.

Blown Glass Containers

The blown glass container process begins by melting the glass components in a refractory furnace at about 1500°C. From the furnace, the glass is poured across a forehearth, where it is cooled to increase its viscosity. It then flows into a hemispherical bowl and out the bottom through holes where the streams are cut into gobs by rotating knives. These gobs flow through a delivery system into the forming machines, which are of two types: blow-blow and press-blow.

Blow-Blow

In blow-blow machines, as shown in Figure 5.1, the gobs fall freely into the mold blank and are pushed by air pressure into the bottom around a plunger which forms the neck and the finish. Then the top of the mold is closed and air is blown upwards through the plunger to simultaneously force the glass outwards against the sides of the mold and form the inner cavity. These steps form a partially shaped object that is called a *parison*. The parison is then inverted and placed in the bottle mold, more heat is added, and air is again blown in to force the gob into the final container shape.

Press-Blow

In the press-blow process, illustrated in Figure 5.2, the gob again drops freely into the mold and then a plunger forces the glass against the mold walls to form the neck and finish. The parison is then inverted, reheated, and air is blown in to push the gob out against the mold cavity.

Traditionally, the blow-blow process has been used for narrow-necked containers and the press-blow process for wide-necked containers. Fundamentally the press-blow process is a better one since it makes container walls that are more uniform and thus can be made thinner, which saves weight and cuts cost. This important advantage led engineers to improve the press-blow process to make it easier to use for narrow-necked containers as well.

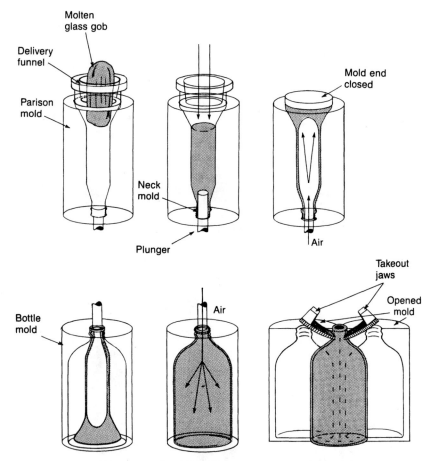

FIGURE 5.1. The blow-blow process simplified.

Annealing and Finishing

The newly formed containers are then transferred to a lehr—an annealing oven—where they are reheated and then very slowly cooled to relieve residual stresses.

After annealing, surface treatments are applied. On the interior surface, SO_2 is blown in where it reacts with Na_2O to form Na_2SO_4 which can be washed off. This makes the surface more resistant to chemical attack. Alternatively, Na_2O can be immobilized by treating the interior surface with fluorohydrocarbon gases.

The outside surface is primed with tin or titanium chlorides

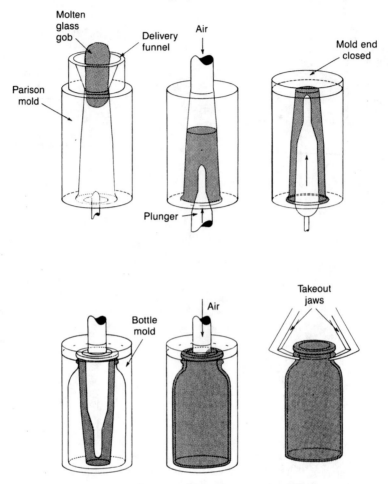

FIGURE 5.2. The press-blow process simplified.

that form a metal oxide layer which is then coated with waxes, stearates, or silicones to reduce the coefficient of friction. Glass container surfaces can be strengthened by putting them in compression. This is accomplished by reacting the container surface with molten potassium salts to convert Na_2O to K_2O at the surface. The larger potassium ion puts the entire surface in compression.

Modern facilities can make up to 300 units/min by the blown glass process.

Ampules and Vials from
Tubular Glass

To make ampules, tubing is heated and pulled in three steps to form the stem, the constriction, and the bulb. The ampule is then trimmed to length, glazed, treated (as above) if necessary, annealed, and packed.

Vials are formed from tubing by heating and pulling off a section which is then rotated while hot against a series of dies to form the finish and the bottom. The finish must be formed to very close tolerances so the elastomeric plug will fit well. The finished vials are then annealed, treated, and packed.

The Fabrication of Metal Containers

Metal containers are generally of two types: two-piece seamless or three-piece welded.

Two-Piece Seamless

Seamless metal containers are made by drawing. This is a process wherein the desired shape is pressed out of a sheet by forcing the sheet into a die. Shallow drawn containers can be made either round or rectangular. Rounds are used for viscous ointments or creams that are hard to squeeze out of a tube. Rectangulars are used for discrete items like tablets or Band-aids. Deep drawn containers are made in a series of drawing steps interspersed with annealing steps. Metal containers with length-to-diameter ratios as high as 14:1 can be made by this method.

An alternative to drawing, used only for soft metals like aluminum, is extrusion. A disc-shaped slug of metal is held in a die and struck with a punch that has the same form as the inside of the finished container. Metal flows against the die bottom and along the outside of the punch. Excess is removed by a stripper plate. The slug thickness determines the eventual wall thickness while the clearance between the punch and the die bottom controls the base thickness, enabling the two to be different. Extrusion can be used for parallel-sided containers of any cross sectional geometry. Restricted apertures and openings, such as narrow necks, can be created by spinning in the open end.

When extrusion is used for collapsible tubes, the slugs are rings that are forced downwards into the die to form the tube shoulder and open nozzle and up around the punch to form the tube wall. The tubes are then cut to length and the nozzle is threaded. After internal coating with vinyl, epoxy, wax, or lacquers, the tube is capped, filled with product through the unconstricted open end, folded, and crimped closed.

Extrusion is also used to make tubes from softer metals such as tin, which, although expensive, is used for some eye medications where maximum inertness is essential.

Whether made by drawing or extrusion, the two-piece metal container is supplied open to the packager who fills it and then applies the top.

Three-Piece Cans

The three-piece can process is more versatile and also more expensive on a per-can basis than the two-piece drawing or extrusion process. It starts with a coil of metal which is cut into sheets that are sometimes then coated. The sheets are slit into rectangular blanks that are bent into cylinders and seamed by soldering or welding. Since these joining processes destroy the coating, it must be repaired as the next step. The can is then completed by flanging both ends, and then seaming the bottom in place. The finished cans, with ends to be applied by the packager, are packed and shipped.

The Fabrication of Plastic Containers

There are four basic types of plastic containers for pharmaceuticals: bottles and vials, blister and strip packages, pouches, and collapsible tubes.

Bottles and Vials

These are made by a blow molding process that resembles the process used for glass bottles but differs from it in several key respects. Most plastic bottles are extrusion blow molded, but the smaller bottles and vials used for most pharmaceuticals are usually injection blow molded, a process which is scrap-free and can produce objects with the accurate neck finish detail that is important for drug containers, particularly vials for parenterals and bottles that require a complex neck finish to accommodate special tamper evident features.

In the injection blow molding process, plastic resin is fed to a rotating screw in a heated barrel, where it is melted and mixed. The resulting hot plastic is then injected at high pressure into a parison cavity around a core rod. The hot parison, shaped more or less like a test tube, is then transferred on the core rod to the bottle mold cavity where it is expanded to fill the cavity by means of air forced in through the core rod.

In practice, injection blow molding machines consist of at least three stations: injection, blowing, and part removal. A typical machine is shown in Figure 5.3.

In extrusion blow molding, molten resin is extruded as a parison into free space and captured by the two halves of a bottle mold. A blow pin is inserted, allowing air pressure to expand the parison against the walls of the mold cavity. After cooling, waste resin must be trimmed from the container bottom. For small containers, such as those used for most drugs, the waste becomes an appreciable fraction of the total container weight, making injection blow molding more efficient for these sizes. HDPE jugs used

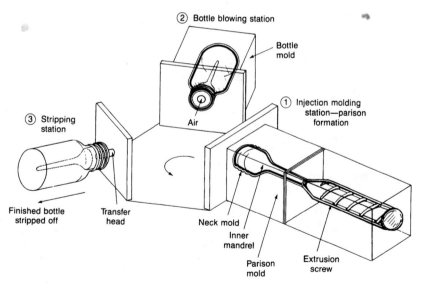

FIGURE 5.3. Three-station injection blow molding machine.

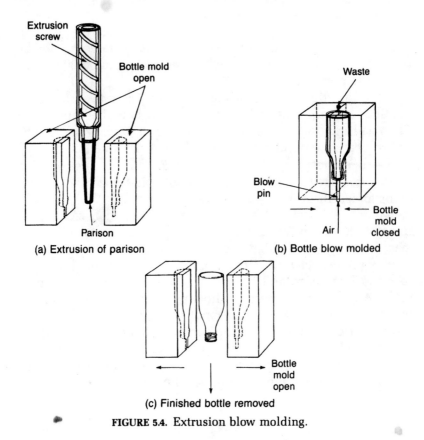

FIGURE 5.4. Extrusion blow molding.

for large quantities of liquids purchased by pharmacies are extrusion blow molded, partly because the handles required on these larger and more awkward containers can be most readily made by that process. Figure 5.4 illustrates a complete extrusion blow molding sequence for a continuous blow molding machine. Note the source of waste illustrated in step (b).

Blister and Strip Packages

These two closely related package types are made in much the same way. The term *blister* is generally reserved for those package types that have a semirigid thermoformed cavity, while *strip* implies a smaller, more flexible, less well-defined cavity. These distinctions will not be rigorously observed in this discussion or in later sections of this book.

Pharmaceutical blister packages are of two basic types:

- those in which clear thermoformed plastic, always PVC or multilayer structures based on PVC, forms the cavity and clear plastic or plastic/paper/foil combinations form the lid
- those that have foil as an essential component of both webs and in which the cavity is created by cold stretching

Although empty preformed blisters and lidding material can be purchased and filled with product in a separate step, this is rarely done. Instead, the package is created and filled on the same machine, as illustrated in Figure 5.5.

The formable web in the case of pharmaceuticals is either plain 5–10 mil PVC or multilayer structures consisting of PVDC-coated PVC, PVC laminated to ACLAR or PVDC film, or PVC laminated to LDPE film. The structures that contain ACLAR or PVDC are used when the product is highly sensitive to moisture or (less often) to oxygen. Since ACLAR-containing structures are several times more expensive than PVDC-containing structures and do not provide any improvement in barrier over PVDC, it is difficult to rationalize their use, other than for reasons of tradition and the desire to be "super-safe."

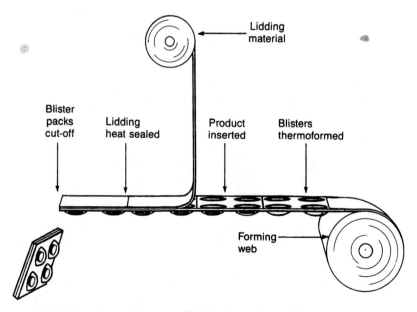

FIGURE 5.5. A continuous roll-fed thermoform-fill-seal machine.

The structure containing LDPE is used when it is important that PVC not contact the product, usually a liquid, or where the superior seal properties of LDPE are required, as with greasy or oily products.

The upper web, or lidding, can be clear plastic but in pharmaceutical packaging is either plain or printed 1-mil foil, for push-through blister types, or paper/foil or paper/PET/foil laminations for the more child-resistant peel-push types.

The formable web is first heated and then drawn across an array of heated dies into which it is forced by vacuum alone, by vacuum plus a male die (plug) assist or by compressed air. After forming and cooling, the blister cavities are filled with product and the lidding, fed off a separate roll, is heat sealed to the sheet of filled cavities. Labeling, notching and perforation, if needed, are then carried out and the continuous roll of lidded blisters is subsequently separated into sheets which typically contain from 10 to 20 individual blisters. Blister machines typically operate with intermittent motion, the seal made during the dwell time required for thermoforming. Line speeds of 200 blisters per minute are achievable with state-of-the-art equipment and readily formable webs such as PVC.

When foil is present in both layers, the structure of the layers is plastic film/adhesive/foil/adhesive/PVC or PE. The outer film, which can be PET or PVC, serves to support the thin aluminum layer. The latter usually consists of several very thin layers rather than a single thicker one since many layers decrease the likelihood of a pinhole passing all the way through and also facilitate the cold stretching process. PVC or PE serve as the heat seal layer. These multilayer webs are formed, filled and sealed on a machine which performs these functions in sequence much as does the thermoform-fill-seal machine pictured in Figure 5.5 except that neither web is heated prior to the forming step.

Modern thermoform-fill-seal machines can be operated at speeds as high as 800 packages/minute.

Plastic Pouches, Bottles, and Make-Fill-Seal Technology

Like bottles and other containers, plastic pouches can be made in one step and then filled in a separate step. Alternatively, both plastic pouches and plastic bottles can be made and filled in the same operation.

Plastic Pouches

The make-fill-seal machines used for pouches are operated in either a horizontal or a vertical configuration. When pouches are made for filling in a separate step, the horizontal machine is used. Figure 5.6 illustrates a horizontal machine set up for packaging a product on the pouch machine. For separate filling, the top seal step is eliminated and the open pouches are picked off and shipped to the filling location where they are filled and heat sealed.

Figure 5.7 shows a vertically oriented form-fill-seal machine. Vertical filling is widely used for dry, free-flowing food products but more rarely for pharmaceuticals.

The vertical machine for making pouches to be filled off-line is shown in Figure 5.8.

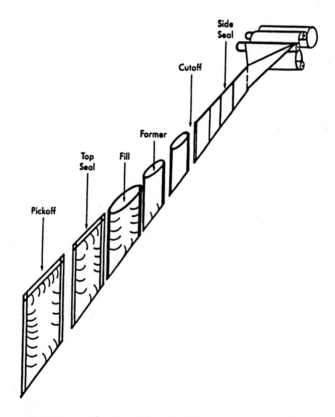

FIGURE 5.6. A horizontal make-fill-seal pouch machine.

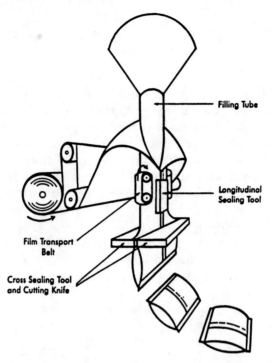

FIGURE 5.7. A vertical form-fill-seal machine.

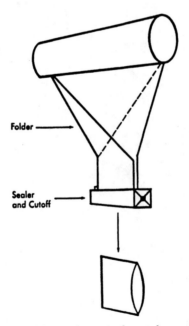

FIGURE 5.8. A vertical pouch machine.

154

The reader who is interested in the details of design and operation of these and other packaging machines used with flexible webs is urged to consult the extensive series of manuals published by the Packaging Machinery Manufacturer's Institute (2000 K St., Washington, DC 20006).

Plastic Bottles by Make-Fill-Seal
Technology

The advent of make-fill-seal machines designed to make, fill and seal plastic pouches in one operation with dry, free-flowing products soon led to the development of analogous machines that could blow, fill and seal plastic bottles in one operation with liquid products. Unlike the make-fill-seal process for dry products which is widely used for foods and other consumer products, the blow-fill-seal process for liquids is used mainly for pharmaceuticals, where it offers an excellent way of maintaining product sterility. Modern blow-fill-seal machines can produce packaged sterile products in a series of aseptic steps that are conducted automatically, without human intervention, in an unbroken sterile environment within the machine itself. Additionally, the packager can avoid the trouble and expense of maintaining a pre-made bottle inventory that must be sterilized before use. Blow-fill-seal containers can range in size from 0.1 ml for ear, nose, and eye drops to 10 liters for irrigation and infusion solutions.

Schematic diagrams of the process are shown in Figures 5.9 and 5.10.

The liquid product to be filled is prepared in sterilized equipment by standard methods and delivered to the machine via a bacteria-retaining filter through sterilized piping. Also fed to the machine are plastic granules (LDPE, HDPE, PP or PE/PP copolymers). The granules are heated and extruded in a mold to form a parison, just as in conventional blow molding [Figure 5.10(a)]. The mold closes around the parison, sealing it at the base and cutting it free at the top. A mandrel unit consisting of two concentric tubes enters the partially formed neck and delivers sterile filtered air through the outer tube which presses the parison against the mold walls while the inner tube delivers a metered volume of sterile filtered solution [Figure 5.10(b)]. After filling, the mandrel retracts and the head mold section closes to seal the container [Figure 5.10(c)]. The mold then opens, releasing the package [Figure 5.10(d)].

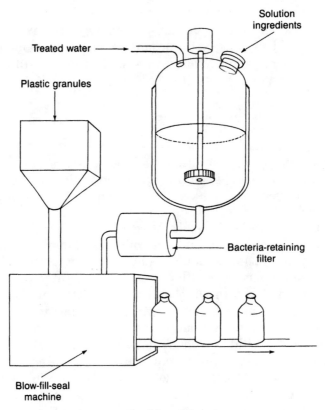

FIGURE 5.9. The blow-fill-seal process.

The necks of the bottles can be molded with screw threads and caps later applied that have additional tamper evident features and devices for breaking the integral container seal immediately before use. One such device, shown in Figure 5.11, uses a cone pin both to pierce the seal and to reseal the opened container.

The plastic granules fed to the machine are not sterile but are unlikely to support microbial growth. Extrusion at 200°C ensures final sterility of this component. As noted, the container is molded by sterile filtered air and positive pressure is maintained at all times within the system. Thus this process offers a high degree of assurance that its products will be sterile until use. To validate this conclusion, experiments have been performed in which foreign matter and bacteria were added to the plastic granule stream. The end products were free of all foreign matter and

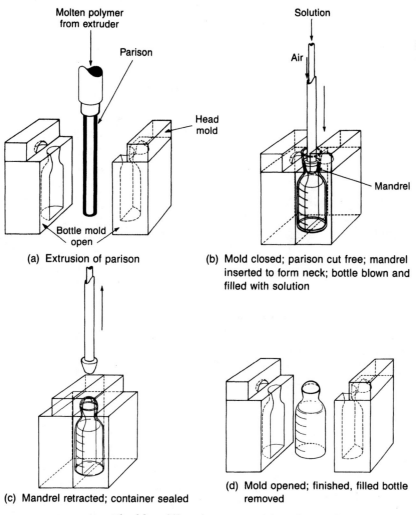

(a) Extrusion of parison

(b) Mold closed; parison cut free; mandrel inserted to form neck; bottle blown and filled with solution

(c) Mandrel retracted; container sealed

(d) Mold opened; finished, filled bottle removed

FIGURE 5.10. The blow-fill-seal process within the machine.

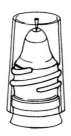

FIGURE 5.11. Cone-pin resealable closure.

157

bacteria. Additional, more rigorous tests have confirmed that this system does an excellent job of preparing sterile products [1].

Collapsible Plastic Tubes

These are of two types: single layer tubes that are coated to enhance appearance and gas barrier, and laminated tubes that contain aluminum foil that provides barrier properties far superior to the coated single layer tube. Tubes are made in two steps — sleeve making and heading.

Single Layer Tubes

The sleeve which forms the body of a single layer tube is made by extruding the plastic resin, commonly LDPE, through a tubing die to form a 14–18 mil wall continuous tube called a *sleeve*. As the hot sleeve emerges from the tubing die, it is exposed to an electric discharge to enhance printing ink adhesion and drawn over a chilled mandrel where it is cooled with a water spray. As the sleeve comes off the mandrel, it is cut to length with a rotary knife. The separated sleeve is printed and then roller-coated with various coatings that impart high gloss and increase the vapor barrier about tenfold.

Heading, the process that attaches the threaded, conically shaped top that carries the closure, is carried out by two methods.

In the Strahm heading process, shown in Figure 5.12, the top end of the sleeve is inserted into the bottom of an injection molding cavity into which molten heading plastic is injected through the top from a low pressure extruder. The molten head is held in contact with the top of the sleeve by the tooling so that it makes a tight fusion seal before it cools. After cooling, excess material is trimmed from above the threaded section, a cap is applied, and the finished tube is packed for shipping to the filler.

In the Downs heading process, shown in Figure 5.13, the sleeve, carried on a tool, enters a punch which is positioned above a strip of hot LDPE. The sleeve is moved down until it is flush with the cutting edge of the punch, and then both drop down, allowing the punch to cut a disc from the LDPE strip which immediately welds to the top edge of the sleeve. The entire mass is then moved to another station where a tool closes on the sleeve and head disc, molding the latter into the final shape. This process eliminates the trim step of the Strahm process.

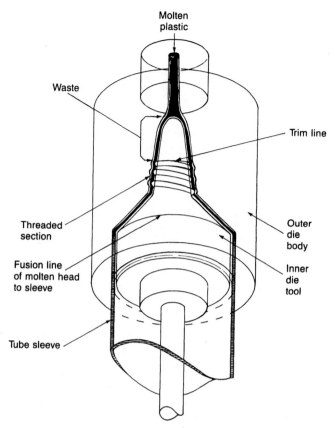

FIGURE 5.12. Creating the head by the Strahm process.

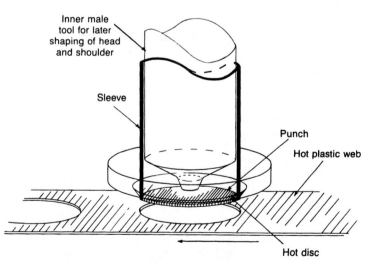

FIGURE 5.13. Heading by the Downs process.

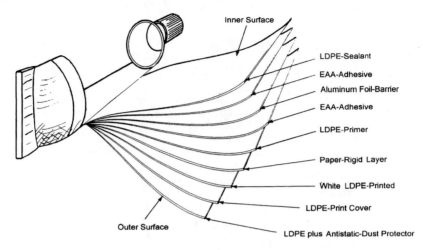

Inner Surface

LDPE-Sealant

EAA-Adhesive

Aluminum Foil-Barrier

EAA-Adhesive

LDPE-Primer

Paper-Rigid Layer

White LDPE-Printed

LDPE-Print Cover

Outer Surface

LDPE plus Antistatic-Dust Protector

FIGURE 5.14. The structure of a typical laminated tube.

Laminated Tubes

Since the laminated tube construction contains paper and aluminum foil, as shown in Figure 5.14, the sleeve cannot be extruded. Instead, it is made by forming the laminated web into a tube and heating the overlapped joint under pressure to seal it closed. The presence of aluminum foil allows induction heating, which can be closely controlled, to be used in the seaming step.

To take advantage of the high barrier properties of the sleeve, an insert made of polybutylene terephthalate, which has good barrier and high temperature properties, is placed above the sleeve in the Strahm heading process and is locked into position by the molten head plastic as it bonds to the sleeve [2].

CONTAINER FILLING AND STERILIZATION

Container Filling

Rigid container filling is usually carried out as a distinct process separate from container making. In contrast, flexible packages, such as blisters and pouches, are almost always filled as part of a form-fill-seal process. Since form-fill-seal processes were covered in the first section of this chapter, only the filling of rigid containers will be described here. The basic steps in the filling operation are essentially the same for all containers. These steps are discussed in some detail for bottles and jars and then variations particular to other containers are covered.

Filling Bottles and Jars

The following basic elements of the filling process are the same for glass and plastic bottles and jars:

- loading the bottles onto a feed or reservoir table
- feeding the bottles into a track which aligns them single file and carries them through subsequent steps
- removing loose foreign matter from inside the bottles
- filling the bottles as they pass under a nozzle or tube
- applying a closure system
- attaching a label
- cartoning, singly or in groups

A generalized filling process is shown in Figure 5.15. In modern, high speed, fully automated lines these steps are carried out in sequence and a variety of devices are employed to correct bottle feed problems without interruption. For example, as bottles are fed onto the conveyer track, the detection of an empty slot signals the filling valve to remain closed as that slot passes under it. Another device identifies bottles that have fallen over or are inverted, and these are automatically removed. Finally, critical steps are validated either by operator observation and record keeping or automatically by detection devices.

Filling with Solids

For powders it is difficult to attain an accurate fill weight since flow is irregular. As a result, broader tolerances in content are permitted. For automated filling, granules are preferred since they flow freely. Control of the fill is generally accomplished by filling cavities which have been calibrated to deliver the desired weight of product. In a typical filling machine for sterile powders, a wheel rim contains cavities which fit precisely and tightly under the filling nozzle when the cavities are in the top position of the wheel. A vacuum helps assure a complete fill and holds the

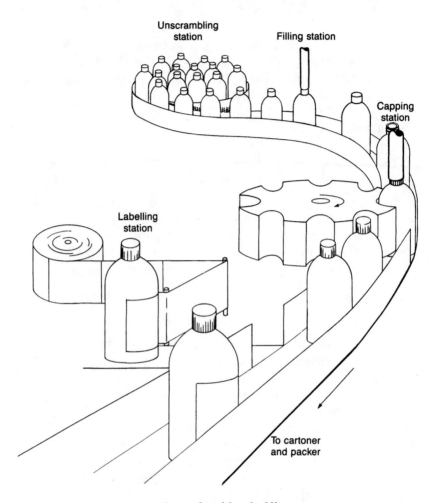

FIGURE 5.15. Generalized bottle filling process.

powder in place as the wheel rotates 180 degrees to the container filling station. At this point, the vacuum is broken and air is used to force the powder into the container. This process is shown in Figure 5.16. Another filling device employs an auger in the stem of a funnel and regulates the fill by controlling the size of the auger and speed of rotation.

For tablet filling, exact tablet count is achieved by highly versatile electronic or mechanical counting machines that can handle tablets and capsules over a range of sizes at rates up to 40,000 per minute by filling seven containers at a time. Despite the high accuracy of tablet counters, check weighing of filled bottles is also employed (see liquid filling). These operations are followed by insertion of cushioning material, capping and the application of a label.

Validation for each of the critical steps is carried out in different ways. At filling speeds of 100 bottles per minute, operators can observe discrepancies. For high speed machines (300 bottles per minute) sensing devices must be used. For example, the absence of a cotton wad, foil inner seal, cap or label can all be detected and the defective package automatically removed from the line. Methods for validating the correctness of the label are described in Chapter Seven. Finally, where cartons are used, sensors can identify an empty carton and remove it.

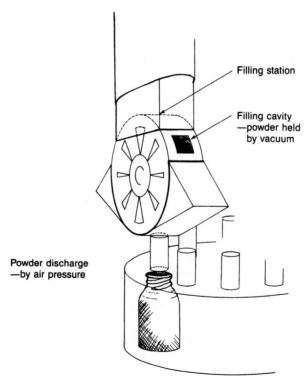

FIGURE 5.16. Rotary machine for powder filling.

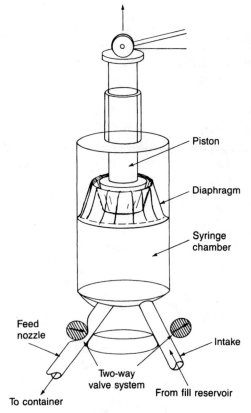

FIGURE 5.17. Piston pump with diaphragm for liquid filling.

Filling with Liquids and Semisolids

For filling small containers, control of content is achieved by regulating the volume of liquid as it is delivered into the container using a pump, or pressure and a valve. One type of pump is a syringe. For automated delivery, a motor drives the piston in continuous strokes and a two way valve allows liquid to be drawn into the syringe chamber on the upstroke and forced out of the feed nozzle on the downstroke. In Figure 5.17, a piston pump is shown that includes a diaphragm to separate the liquid from the piston. Other kinds of pumps include an auger turning in the stem of a funnel and a pulsating diaphragm. When the flow of liquid is driven by the pressure of gas in the head space of the feed tank, an on-off valve controls the fill volume. One example of such a valve is a flexible tube which is pinched off using a mechanically driven clamp or pinch roll. A diagram of such a filling system is shown in Figure 5.18. For large containers, the fill is regulated by filling to a level indicator placed within the container which controls the flow of liquid.

To insure fill accuracy, a number of techniques are used. For the most advanced systems, an accuracy of ± 0.1–0.2% can be achieved. In the case of piston driven pumps and diaphragm pumps activated by pistons, precise adjustment of the piston

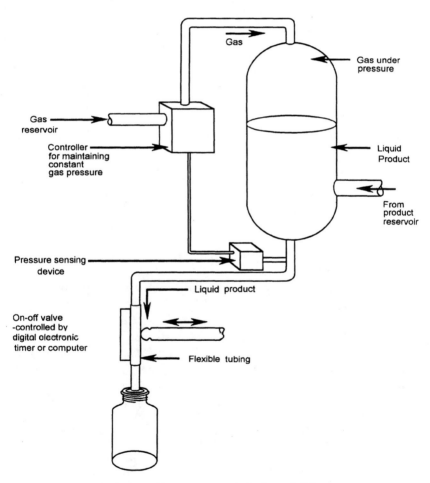

FIGURE 5.18. Pressure system for liquid filling.

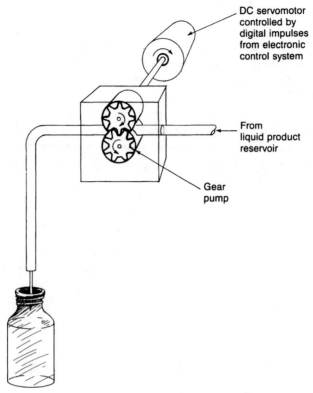

FIGURE 5.19. Precision gear pump system for liquid filling.

stroke is the key. For motor driven screws or augers, control of the number of revolutions must be extremely accurate. The highest level of accuracy is achieved in a unit that utilizes a positive displacement gear pump driven by a DC servomotor which is in turn controlled by digital impulses from an electronic control system (see Figure 5.19). For the pressurized tank and valve system, the head space gas pressure is adjusted to compensate for changing volume so that constant pressure is maintained. Accurate electronic timers determine the duration of the filling cycle. Even with the most precise control of volume fill, check weighers are also employed. Typically, some or all of the containers rest on load cells which feed the weights of empty and filled containers into computers that keep the tare and final weights sorted out and calculate net fill weights. In some machines, fill weights are used directly to control the filling cycle by feeding electronic signals to either control the duration of a valve opening (e.g., for a pressurized feed tank), or the length of a piston stroke or the number of revolutions of a screw pump [3].

In all of these techniques for liquid filling, the filling tube is inserted well into the neck of the bottle to avoid spillage. The diameters of the filling tube and of the bottle neck must be matched to achieve the desired filling rate. The filling tube must be small enough to permit the ready escape of air from the bottle as it is filled. Larger diameter filling tubes allow higher filling rates and are necessary for viscous liquids.

Filling with Sterile Liquids

In filling glass ampules with sterile liquids, very small diameter filling tubes are used because of the narrow neck. Before the tube is withdrawn after filling, a mechanism draws the droplet on the tip back into the tube to avoid wetting the neck. Once filled, the ampules are sealed using hot gas-oxygen flames to soften and melt the neck. To insure uniform heating, the ampules are either rotated in a single flame or are surrounded by several flames. The seals are made by allowing the molten glass to collapse on itself forming a bead or by pulling and twisting closed the soft neck as shown in Figure 5.20. Sealing is quicker using the bead method but closure is more certain in the twist procedure. The twist seal must be used for wider mouthed ampules to avoid the thermal strains in a large bead which could lead to cracking. These operations are mechanized in automated filling machines.

For vials and bottles, precisely controlled volumes of parenteral liquids are introduced automatically. Because of the larger mouth, larger diameter filling tubes are used, making this a much easier process than for ampules. The elastomeric closures are pushed into the filled container using a plunger and aluminum caps are then fitted over the stopper and crimped under the lip of the vial or bottle. To prefill syringes, the cleaned, siliconized and sterilized syringes and plungers are separately fed to different positions on the filling line. The syringes, with or without needles in place, are fitted with a protective cap, inverted and indexed to a two-position head where first they are filled and then the plunger is inserted to the predetermined fill line. After inspection, the filled syringes are automatically placed into cartons.

Inspection of all packaged parenteral liquids is necessary to de-

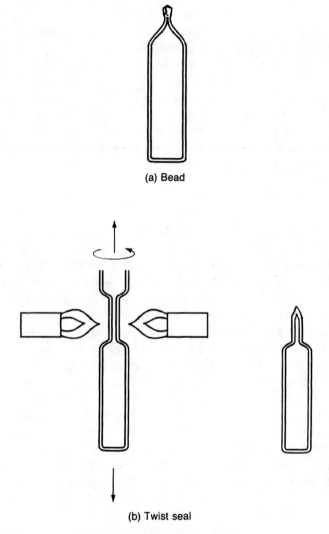

(a) Bead

(b) Twist seal

FIGURE 5.20. Sealing of ampules.

tect the presence of particulates. This can be done automatically. In one unit, the images of the solutions are projected onto a number of highly sensitive photo-sensors which transmit the detection of floating particulates to electronic circuitry which triggers the automatic rejection of the package prior to cartoning. The unit detects under- or over-filled containers as well.

Filling Collapsible Tubes

Collapsible metal tubes are produced with the tops capped and sealed and the bottoms left open to their full diameter for filling. Fully mechanized tube packaging lines consist of four steps: tube feeding, cleaning, filling and closing. In a typical high speed operation, tubes are fed from a chute and rolled into a magazine section where a tool insures a tight fitting cap. Compressed air is used to blow particles out of the tube. The tubes are then raised to a vertical position for filling from a metering device such as a volumetric piston pump. After filling, the ends are flattened and sealed (usually with a double fold) and crimped. Sealants based on vinyls, lacquers or latex are sometimes applied to improve the gas barrier of the crimp. Plastic tubes are filled similarly and the bottoms heat sealed. Laminated tubes can be sealed using ultrasonic equipment which substantially lowers the cost of converting filling lines for metal tubes to plastic. For soft metal tubes, a carton is usually necessary for protection, and insertion of the finished tube into the carton is the last step in the packaging line.

Filling Aerosol Containers

The basic steps for filling aerosol containers are similar to those for bottles but are modified to accommodate the special needs of pressurized containment. The fully fabricated cans, with an opening in the top for the valve, are aligned and fed to a conveyer line where they are cleaned and indexed to a station where the several loading functions are performed automatically. These include the loading of an agitator ball if required, filling with liquid or powdered ingredients, inserting the preassembled valve, crimping the valve assembly in place, evacuating air from the container and charging in the propellant through the valve. An alternative is to charge the propellant under the valve cap followed by crimping to secure the valve. Under-the-cap charging is accomplished by employing a crimping bell that creates a temporary seal around the top of the container so that air can be evacuated and propellant added followed by seating and crimping of the valve cap, all within the bell. Charging under the cap is faster since a larger opening is available.

Although the propellant is usually charged in under pressure at room temperature, for nonaqueous products it can be chilled to

$-40°F$ and added to the prechilled container and contents. Initially the cold filling method allowed higher production speeds, but advances in pressure filling have led to comparable filling rates and pressure filling is now more common. Once filled and closed, the aerosol container is tested either by vacuum or in a bath to assure a completely sealed system.

Both straight line and rotary filling lines are used. For straight line filling, cans are usually carried in plastic supports or pucks and moved intermittently so that a set of filling/valving/crimping/charging stations operates simultaneously on one group of cans at a time. The output is approximately doubled for lines that contain two sets of stations. The production rate for straight line machines is 20 to 150 cans per minute. Rotary machines, where cans are positioned on the periphery of a wheel, feature more positive can control, increased productivity and access to the bottom of the can for coding. For high speed rotary machines, all operations (charging, crimping, etc.) are driven by rotary action and are continuous. Such machines can fill as many as 300 aerosol cans per minute. When flammable propellants are used, the charging station must be remotely located in an explosion-proof environment.

Validation of aerosol performance consists of testing critical parts, measuring and verifying contents and demonstrating functions critical to therapeutic effectiveness. One of the more critical parts is the metered dose valve. Validation of dose delivery is established by discharging standard test solutions through standard actuators for fixed time periods and measuring the dose delivered by weight loss of the aerosol. Among the factors important to therapeutic effectiveness is the spray pattern. This can be measured by spraying the aerosol onto paper treated with a dye-talc mixture. Dyes are selected that are soluble in the aerosol contents so that droplets cause the dye to be absorbed into the paper and to reveal the spray pattern. The particle size distribution of the droplets, critical for respiratory aerosols, is measured in several ways. In one of the most popular, the aerosol passes through a series of nozzles, striking impact plates arranged so that the largest particles are collected first and the smallest last. Light scattering techniques are also used in which the varying intensity of a light beam is measured as an aerosol settles under turbulent conditions.

Sterile Packaging

In Chapter Two the problem of microorganisms and pyrogens for both nonsterile and sterile pharmaceuticals was described and the general approaches for their control were discussed. Here, the specific processes used for sterilization and the integration of these processes into the filling operation will be covered.

The preferred technique is terminal sterilization of the final packaged product as soon as possible after sealing. Where terminal sterilization is not possible because of drug sensitivity to the sterilization conditions, the pharmaceutical is aseptically packaged in equipment where the product and the package are separately sterilized and then brought together in a sterile environment. For critical products, such as parenterals, aseptic packaging is combined with terminal sterilization. For noncritical products, aseptic packaging is often used even though terminal sterilization is possible.

Terminal Sterilization

Autoclaving with saturated steam under pressure is the most common terminal sterilization method. For large scale operations, assemblages of packages are placed in the autoclave, which is a thick-walled steel pressure vessel. The periods for heating up, holding at sterilization conditions and for cooling down are regulated to suit the heat sensitivity of the package and the drug and the time required to achieve the required level of microorganism destruction. For especially sensitive products, like dextrose for injection, the heating rate is very rapid and cooling is accelerated by water sprays. Autoclaving is used primarily for aqueous liquids. It is ineffective for dry powders in sealed containers and anhydrous oils.

For materials such as petroleum jelly, mineral oils, greases, waxes and talcum powder, where steam sterilization is ineffective or is too severe, filled packages are subjected to dry heat in a hot air oven. A wide range of inactivation times and temperatures have been established which depend on the bacteria involved and the humidity. Lower temperature cycles have been developed for some preparations such as sulfonamides, powders with low melting points and certain oil-based solutions which cannot withstand normal conditions.

Nonthermal methods of sterilization that are commonly employed for medical devices are not generally suitable for pharmaceuticals, especially liquids, since ionizing radiation adversely affects the drug and sterilizing gases will not penetrate the package. An exception is the European practice of using ionizing radiation to sterilize some powders, such as penicillin, streptomycin, polyvitamins and certain hormones. While no drugs are sterilized this way in the U.S., several drug/container systems are presently in the FDA approval process. It is predicted that in the future, radiation will be used for final sterilization once a drug has been aseptically packaged. These radiation doses will be considerably smaller than those required for primary sterilization thus avoiding radiation damage to drugs and packaging materials [4].

Aseptic Packaging

Aseptic packaging requires separate sterilization of the equipment, the product, the package, and the environment. The necessity for sterilizing the package is illustrated by the experience with unsterilized brick pack cartons where microorganism counts as high as 40 per carton have been recorded [5]. The containers may be supplied to the drug packager already cleaned and sterilized, or they may be cleaned and sterilized in the aseptic filling line, or the containers may be manufactured under conditions that insure sterility as part of the filling operation, as in the case of plastic containers in make-and-fill processes.

The sequence of steps for preparing containers that are free of particulates and microorganisms usually includes washing, drying, sterilization and cooling. For in-line sterilization of glassware, containers are commonly exposed to a laminar flow of very hot air (as high as 350°C) while being passed through a Class 100 tunnel. Such a tunnel contains, per cubic foot of air, less than 100 particles 0.5 microns or larger in size. Generally, a container temperature of 180–200°C is sufficient for achieving sterility and contact time if the oven is adjusted to account for container size and shape. The air used is recycled, filtered and dried if containers are wet from washing. Upon emerging from the tunnel, containers are cooled with filtered laminar flow air washed over an area in a stable layer isolating the area from the surrounding environment and controlling the level of airborne particles.

Autoclaving is also used for glassware where lower sterilization temperatures are acceptable (115–138°C) since wet heat is more effective in killing microorganisms than dry heat. These lower temperatures permit the use of autoclaves to sterilize more heat sensitive containers, closures and packages such as those made from plastics including nylon, HDPE, polyesters, PP and elastomers.

Plastic containers are also sterilized using ethylene oxide by placing articles in a chamber containing the gas for four hours at 130°F. Upon completion of sterilization, gas is removed by vacuum and the containers are stored until residual gas and by-products dissipate. This last step is critical since residuals can irritate the skin and mucous membranes. Chemical sterilization by immersion in liquids is widely used for plastics and paper packages in aseptic filling operations. For the Tetra Brik process, which is a make-and-fill operation where a box is formed from a paper, plastic, aluminum foil laminate, the laminate is immersed in a bath of 35% hydrogen peroxide. In this case the residual sterilization products have been shown to be at an acceptably low level or harmless. Collapsible metal tubes are sterilized with dry heat or by autoclaving. Irradiation sterilization of containers and closures has been widely studied but is not used except for medical devices.

Sterilization of liquid products prior to aseptic packaging is accomplished by autoclaving, heating and/or filtration. Filters used must have openings small enough to retain microorganisms and yet allow reasonable flow rates. Pressure or vacuum assist increases the rate of flow. Common filter materials include fused porcelain, sintered glass or metal and cellulosic or plastic membranes. Typically, coarser first stage and finer second stage filters are employed with pore sizes of about 0.3–0.5 and 0.2–0.3 microns for each stage respectively.

A typical sterile operation was recently described for filling blown HDPE bottles with liquids [6]. Isolated Class 100 areas are maintained for the remote bottle making operation and filling steps, while intermediate Class 1000 areas (a cubic foot of air contains no more than 1000 particles 0.5 microns or larger) enclose transition operations such as bottle handling, storage and cartoning. Bottles coming off the blow molding line are packaged in three layers of presterilized polyethylene bags. As the bottles leave the bottle making area, the outer bag is removed. The middle bag is discarded during the transition into the filling area. The final bag is removed just prior to loading bottles into the filling operation. By this technique, contamination from each previous area is left behind at each transition point. The blow molding equipment is designed so that all parts can be cleaned and sterilized including bottles, molds, and conveyor lines. In the filling operation, liquids sterilized by heat and/or filtration are brought together with bottles and presterilized caps to complete the aseptic process.

Some of these elaborate bagging procedures and the Class 1000 handling areas can be eliminated when the bottle blowing operation is carried out immediately adjacent to the filling and sealing steps. In this case, the whole process can be enclosed and fitted with internal sterile air showers so the critical filling point is in an aseptic area and the whole process runs without the need for operator intervention. This isolation of the process from operating personnel eliminates the major source of contamination, according to a recent survey of pharmaceutical companies [7].

Sterilization Validation

Autoclave effectiveness must be validated before new apparatus is put into service using commercially prepared, heat resistant spores. Continued effectiveness is monitored with these same microorganisms combined with measurements of the temperatures by means of thermocouples or indicators that change colors or melt.

For purposes of validating sterility in finished packages of injectables, statistically selected samples of each lot must be tested for sterility. A lot, for autoclaving, is defined as containing packages that have all experienced identical conditions of sterilization. For aseptic filling, a lot constitutes packages produced during no more than a working day or shift and when there was no change in equipment.

In the *USP* procedure for sterility testing, product from sterilized packages is used directly to inoculate culture media, or the liquid product is filtered and washings from the filter are used to inoculate culture media. The recommended media are soybean-casein digest medium and fluid thioglycolate medium. Incubation periods vary from seven to fourteen days and temperatures range from 20° to 35°C depending on the medium and the methods of sterilization and inoculation. Pyrogens are detected by injecting product into rabbits and looking for a fever response or by the Limulus test, in which the product is mixed with a substance that gels or changes color in the presence of pyrogens.

From the analysis of sampling and probability data, it is clear that sterility testing is a poor method of validating sterilization procedures. A better approach is the use of biological indicators such as highly resistant bacterial spores. It is necessary that the bacteria used as an indicator be more numerous and have a greater resistance to sterilization than the microbes expected in the product to be sterilized. There are species of bacteria that are commonly accepted for biological indicators for the various methods of sterilization. These indicators are carried along with the packages being sterilized on either paper or plastic strips or are inoculated into the product being sterilized.

In an aseptic filling operation where the liquid is sterilized by filtration, a liquid media fill can be used which substitutes for the normal pharmaceutical product. The media fill is a liquid that promotes the growth of microorganisms. In a reported example of this procedure, the aseptic line was cleaned in the normal fashion and all monitoring was carried out as for a typical manufacturing run. Liquid tryptone soya medium was added to the initial mix tank, filtered (0.45 microns prefilter and 0.22 microns final filter), pumped through the transfer lines and filtered again (two 0.22 microns filters in series) before entering the form-fill-seal operation. As made, the media fill contained 5000 microorganisms per ml, a significant challenge to the filtration system. Finished packages containing the media fill were incubated and examined for microorganism growth. In addition, some packages were inoculated with *Bacillus subtilis, Staphylococcus aureus* or *Candida albicans* to validate the test. In the initial validation of the equipment, only two packages out of 36,000 showed growth, and these were shown to have been damaged subsequent to filling. The normal recommendation is to incubate at least 3000 units so that there is a 95% probability of detecting a contamination level of 1 in 1000 [7].

REFERENCES

1. Sharp, I. 1987. *Pharm. J.* (July 25):106.
2. Bakker, M., ed. 1986. *The Wiley Encyclopedia of Packaging Technology.* New York, NY: John Wiley & Sons, p. 686.
3. Kelsey, R. J. 1987. *Food and Drug Packaging* (November):8–12.
4. B. Reid, Nordion Corporation, private communication, 1991.
5. Guise, W. 1986. *Manufacturing Chemist* (April):61–64.
6. Holmgren, B. R. 1990. *Packaging* (May):44–49.
7. Sharp, J. 1990. *J. Parenteral Sci. and Technology,* 44(Sept.-Oct.):289–292.

CHAPTER SIX

Closures for
Pharmaceutical Packages

All packages must be closed to protect and contain the contents. Closure is accomplished in one of three ways: sealing the container with adhesives, sealing the container with heat, or by the use of separate devices.

Closures are particularly important in drug packaging because the variety of closures used for drugs is greater than for any other group of commodities and the standards for closure performance are more critical in drug packaging than in any other field. In addition, drug package closure designers and engineers must cope with three factors which are more pervasive, more important and more thoroughly regulated in that field than in any other: child resistance, tamper evidence, and the special needs of the elderly.

This chapter begins with a discussion of the various types of closures used in drug packaging, their functions, the materials they are made from and how they are joined to the container. Closure liners, child resistant closures and tamper evident closures are then treated in subsequent sections.

CLOSURE BY ADHESIVES
OR HEAT SEALING

These two closure techniques are widely used in food and retail goods packaging but much less frequently in drug packages since most drugs are packaged in rigid containers that do not lend themselves to these techniques. Exceptions are the use of adhesives for closing boxes and heat sealing for closing blisters, strip packs, ampules and plastic tubes. Since boxes are not the primary packages with which this book is concerned, the subject of adhesive closures will not be dealt with further. Heat sealing is treated elsewhere in connection with blister packages, ampules and tubes.

Not all flexible containers need be heat sealed or closed by adhesives. Bags and drum liners can be tied with string or wire-reinforced plastic strips. If the top of the bag is twisted and then folded over on itself, a secure, liquid-tight closure can be effected, but the vapor barrier is inferior to that obtained by heat or adhesive sealing.

CLOSURE BY SEPARATE DEVICES

This section deals with the separate closure devices used for cans, bottles, jars, vials, and tubes. Closure of aerosol containers is treated in Chapter Five.

Closure Functions

Protective Containment

This is the most important closure function. *Containment* requires that the contents not escape through the closure until they are needed by the consumer. *Protective* means that external factors such as moisture, gases or other contaminants are kept away from the packaged product and that the closure not interact with the drug contents in any way that would alter the purity, potency or efficacy of the product.

Positive Sealing

This function is closely related to protective containment. It requires that when the closure is applied, continuous contact is achieved between the inside top of the closure and either the top lip of the container, if the closure is a cap, or the finish bead and the inside of the container neck, if the container is a vial. The use of closure liners to assist in this function is described in the next section.

Access

This is the most difficult function for any closure to perform. The ideal drug package closure, while first providing the essential function of protective containment, must also:

- for OTC drugs, provide an obvious signal if it has been tampered with
- for prescription drugs and certain OTC drugs, pass the child-resistant closure (CRC) requirements and also be easily openable by the elderly and infirm
- be easily reclosable
- in the case of parenteral vials, be penetrable by a needle many times without allowing that action to expose the vial contents to contamination

Fortunately for closure designers, this last requirement, which can be met only by elastomeric materials, need never be coupled with the tamper evidence and CRC requirements.

Communication and Display

While the functions of communication and display may not be obvious at first glance, they are nevertheless important considerations in today's closure designs. Specifically, they include:

- The incorporation, on the closure, of directions for opening it—obvious examples are the wording *press down and turn,* or an arrow which must be aligned with another arrow on the container or an arrow which signifies the direction of dispensing in spray-type containers.
- Written material such as the manufacturer's name or logo.
- Styling or identification features: while most prescription drug bottle caps are white, in keeping with the sterility and cleanliness image, OTC drug closures are frequently pastel colored. Different colors may be used for different size containers of the same product, or the color can be carefully coordinated with the container color to provide enhanced aesthetics, particularly for fragrances and cosmetics. Color contrast may also be used to direct the user to the flip-up section of a closure which has this

feature. The ready pigmentability of thermoplastics is one reason for their increasing popularity as closures versus thermosetting plastics or metal.

Types of Separate Device Closures

Cans

Three closure types are used for cans: slip lids, friction lids, and threaded lids.

Slip lids fit over the can top and rely on friction and either a shrink band or pressure sensitive tape to hold them in place. They can be used for semisolids such as pastes and ointments. For solid drugs that are moisture sensitive, a slip lid needs a closure liner to provide a moisture barrier.

Friction lids are far more secure and provide a much better moisture barrier. An example is the common paint can lid, which makes a plug type seal against the rim along the can top.

If a high degree of moisture protection is required, cans are used that have a foil diaphragm at the top which is clinched into the top seam when the friction lid is applied. These containers are supplied to the packager with the friction lid already in place and are filled from the bottom. The bottom end is then spun on after being lined with a resilient material to make a tight seal.

Finally, some cans are made with screw threads at the top to accept the same type of threaded closures discussed in the next section.

Bottles and Jars

Closures for bottles and jars are of two types: threaded and friction-fit.

Threaded Closures

Most drug bottles and jars now have threaded closures. These have replaced corks which were fragile, incompatible with liquid drugs, and could not be sterilized. Threaded closures can be subdivided into three types: continuous-thread, lug, and metal roll-on.

Continuous-Thread (CT)

This closure type is the one most commonly used for drugs. Since the threads on both closure and container form an inclined plane, the application of sufficient torque can generate a very tight seal between the closure and bottle lip. Proper closure torque requires a delicate balance between closure security and the ability of a consumer to readily open the container. Today, capping machines that mechanically apply such closures can be electronically adjusted to apply torque in finite increments and off-line testers can assure that the desired tension is continuously maintained.

Although the efficiency of the seal can be enhanced with a separate liner, many thermoplastic CT closures now employ a variety of molded-in features to allow satisfactory linerless sealing for drugs that *USP* recommends be either "well closed" or "tightly closed."

CT closures are made of aluminum, tinplate, tin-free steel, thermosets and thermoplastics, but for drug packaging, the thermoplastic designs are by far the most common.

One design combines thermoplastics and thermosets—the CT-plug combination illustrated in Figure 6.1.

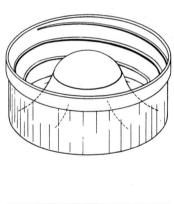

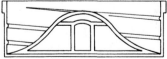

FIGURE 6.1. The CT-plug combination closure.

The cap is a strong, hard thermoset but the conical plug within is a softer thermoplastic. When screwed on with only modest torque, the plug readily conforms to the inside of the bottle neck, making a very effective seal with no tendency to release due to cold flow.

CT closures have one disadvantage: with plastic bottles, they are less secure than with glass bottles. When a CT closure is screwed down on a glass bottle, it meets an unyielding surface, whereas with a plastic bottle, particularly one made of polyethylene, both cap and bottle will slowly deform. This "cold flow" phenomenon causes the release torque to slowly decrease. The use of stiffer thermoplastics, PP, PVC or PET, for both closures and bottles, ameliorates this problem.

Lug

The lug closure also operates on the principle of thread engagement but in this case, only the container is threaded. The thread is interrupted at intervals to allow engagement by two, four, or six lugs on the cap. When the cap is pushed down so the lugs are under the thread, a quarter turn tightly engages the closure (Figure 6.2).

These closures can be installed quickly and removed quickly, making them particularly suitable for high-speed capping lines. Since the design does not allow precise adjustment of application torque, closure liners are frequently used to ensure a tight seal.

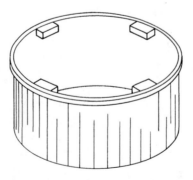

FIGURE 6.2. Lug closure.

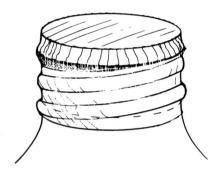

FIGURE 6.3. Roll-on closure.

Metal Roll-On

This style uses thread engagement with a different capping process. An unthreaded blank is placed over the threaded container neck and a combination of downward pressure (to create a tight seal) and rotation of the cap sides against hardened steel dies forces the cap sides to assume the threaded contours of the bottle neck (Figure 6.3).

Only metal has the requisite ductility for this closure method; aluminum is almost universally used for the purpose. Unless a tamper evident feature is incorporated, the lower end of the cap thread must bleed into the transfer ring on the bottle to prevent it from being rolled under this ring and becoming difficult to remove.

Roll-on closures are widely used in food, beverage, and drug packaging. They adapt well to a variety of top pressures which control the tightness of the seal, there is no application torque to worry about, it is a very rapid capping method (speeds in excess of 1220/min are possible) and it is readily adapted to include a tear-off band for tamper evidence.

When the tear-off band is to be incorporated, the bottom edge of the cap blank is perforated and made long enough to be molded under a locking ring at the bottom of the threaded section of the bottle neck. Initial cap removal tears off the bottom section at the perforation, leaving it in place under the locking ring to provide evidence of entry.

Roll-on closures are not used when the bottle contents include syrupy or adhesive liquids. When such liquids dribble over the bottle threads, the cap, when reapplied, will stick and thwart the next attempt to open the container.

Friction-Fit Closures

As the name implies, this closure type relies on friction to hold the cap in place and to provide and sustain enough downward pressure to maintain the seal. There are four basic types: crown, snap-fit, press-on, and stoppers.

Crown Closures

These are the common traditional beverage bottle closures found rarely on drug packages. They are made of tinplate or tin-free steel and are designed with flutes that are created by crimping a blank over the bottle neck on the capping machine (Figure 6.4). Liners are always used with these closures to effect a tight seal.

Snap-Fit Caps

These are pressed on the bottle and held in place by friction or friction plus the engagement of supplementary ridges, flanges or grooves that mate with structures on the outer rim of the bottle. They are always made of plastic and are frequently used on containers for OTC drugs. One variation of this design fits the tamper evident criteria: a cap long enough to be snapped down over a shoulder on the bottle and that can be initially removed only by tearing off a perforated breakaway strip. Another variation is used

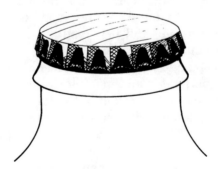

FIGURE 6.4. Crown closure.

as a child-resistant closure by outfitting it with a lug which fits over a matching gap in a ring molded into the container neck. When the cap is rotated, the lug engages the ring and cannot easily be removed. This variation is quite common in prescription drug repackaging by pharmacists.

Press-On Vacuum Caps

This closure system relies on a partial vacuum in the container headspace and a closure liner to create the seal required. Additional security is sometimes gained by forcing the cap over a ridge on the container neck. Press-on vacuum caps are mainly used for oxygen sensitive food products, since few drugs require the tight seal provided by this system.

Stoppers for Vials

Originally made from cork, stoppers for drug containers are now universally made from a variety of elastomeric materials. These materials are discussed in detail in Chapter Four: their composition, structures, methods of manufacture and the way shapes are made from them. Stoppers are the only separate closure suitable for vials containing injectables. No other material, natural or synthetic, will reseal itself after being penetrated by a needle.

Vial stoppers for injectables must meet the following requirements:

- They must reseal after being punctured.
- They must seal the vial in a way that maintains a sterile environment inside it.
- Their interaction with the vial contents must be kept to the lowest level possible.
- They must not shed particles when punctured.
- They must provide the barrier characteristics demanded by the vial contents.
- They must be capable of withstanding autoclaving conditions that will kill pathogens.
- They must be readily insertable into the vial by automatic closure operations.

Four stopper designs are most commonly used for injectable fluid vials:

1. The flanged plug shown in Figure 6.5 that is secured with an aluminum overseal that has a hole in the center as shown in Figure 6.6. The overseal is crimped over the plug by spinning rollers which rotate around the top of the vial or by a rail machine in which the vial rotates against a stationary rail. This design effects a seal by means of the tight fit between the plug and the vial neck and between the flange and the end of the vial. Good contact between flange and vial neck is maintained by the aluminum overseal.

2. A flanged hollow plug which has cutouts along the plug wall is shown in Figure 6.7. These are used for lyophilized drugs. The plug is partially inserted into the vial so the cutout sections allow passage of the water vapor being pumped off the vial contents during freeze-drying. When drying is complete, the plug is pushed home under vacuum and overcapped as above.

3. Vials are stoppered as in #1 or #2 above but fitted with a solid plastic overcap rather than an aluminum overseal that has a hole in the center. The solid overcap keeps the top of the plug clean so that it does not have to be swabbed with alcohol before the needle is inserted. The plastic overcap must be discarded after the first use.

4. A metal cap as in #1 or #2 is lined with an elastomeric disc. These are for the so-called *dentists' vials* that are so small a separate stopper would be too awkward to handle on capping machines. This design makes a poorer seal than the plug designs.

Because of the extreme danger posed by any form of contamination or alteration of drugs injected into the body, and because of the nature of the elastomers that must be used to close containers for injectables, there are several ongoing concerns with these closures.

Sorption is the first concern. Most injectables contain substances added to control bacterial growth: benzyl alcohol, cresol, chloroxylenol, phenol, and many others. If these bacteriostats are sorbed into the closure, their concentration will drop below the effective limit. The most straightforward way of avoiding this

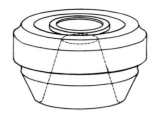

FIGURE 6.5. Flanged plug for vials.

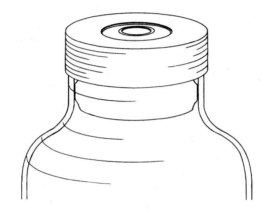

FIGURE 6.6. Aluminum overseal for flanged plug.

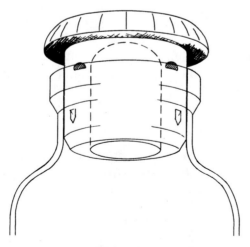

FIGURE 6.7. Flanged cutout plug.

187

problem is to soak the closure in a solution of the bacteriostat to be used before it is inserted into the container. This approach is awkward in practice, so the best way to minimize the problem is through the proper choice of elastomer composition and bacteriostat.

Transfer of elastomer components to the drug product is the next concern. As noted in Chapter Four, it is not uncommon for an elastomeric composition to contain eight to ten nonelastomeric components. Any or all of these may be leached out of the elastomer by an injectable solution. This is one reason why ly-ophilized injectables are used. For liquid injectables, only careful compatibility testing can control the problem.

An elegant way to finesse both sorption and leaching problems is to line the stopper with a thin layer of Teflon® [1], a polymer un-matched in its inertness to chemicals. While this adds cost to the closure, the development of practical techniques for Teflon coating has nevertheless given the packager an excellent way to cure these two problems.

Particulate matter from the closure is always of concern to the packager of injectables. Particulate matter can be broken away from the stopper during penetration or withdrawal of the needle. The incorporation of soft natural rubber in the elastomer formu-lation mitigates this problem. Other sources of particulate matter are particles abraded during washing and fillers released from the elastomer if surface breakdown occurs. Abrasion can be mini-mized by eliminating sharp edges or corners on the stopper and by minimizing violent mechanical agitation in the washing and drying operations. Redeposition of washed off material can be avoided by proper design of the washing operation. Choice of elastomer composition or lining the stopper with Teflon can con-trol filler release.

Closures for Tubes

A collapsible tube has two closures: one that seals the nozzle through which the contents are extruded by the user, and one that seals the open end through which the tube is filled by the manu-facturer.

A CT cap made from metal or plastic is the usual choice for closing the nozzle. The plastic types can be either thermosetting, in which case closure liners are used, or thermoplastic which can be designed to be linerless. An innerseal is often incorporated for tamper evidence and gas barrier. For medications applied through a body cavity, a nozzle integrally molded onto the cap is usually provided, in which case the plastic snap-fit closure is used.

After metal tubes have been filled, the open end is crimped, rolled, and recrimped. The ends of plastic tubes are sealed dielectrically or with heat. This makes an absolutely leak-proof seal that is tamper evident.

Convenience Closures

Recent years have seen closure manufacturers using plastic to create closures which perform all the essential functions described above but are easier to use. Much of this effort has centered on closures for food packaging but has also spilled over into drug packaging.

Fixed-Spout Closures

These closures are fitted with a tubular projection used to dispense the contents at a targeted area, either on the body or on a food product such as hot dogs. The closure itself can be CT or snap-on. If the spout is sealed, the orifice size can be selected by cutting the tapered spout at the proper point. Alternatively, the spout may be closed with a small friction overcap which enables a snip-tip spout to be reclosed.

Movable-Spout Closures

Some of these feature a hinged spout which can be flipped into the open position and then reclosed with one hand (Figure 6.8). A tear band can be affixed across the hinged section to provide tamper evidence. Another design is the push-pull type (Figure 6.9) that is opened and closed by pulling and pushing in a straight line.

Plug-Orifice Flip-Top Closures

These were first introduced for personal care products (Figure 6.10) and were the first closures to utilize the hinged top design made possible by the excellent flex-crack resistance of polypropyl-

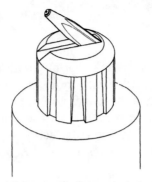

FIGURE 6.8. Flip-spout closure.

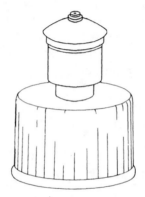

FIGURE 6.9. Push-pull closure.

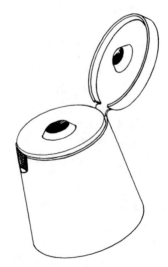

FIGURE 6.10. Hinged plug-orifice closure.

ene. These closures have moved broadly into the packaging of viscous pharmaceuticals. As shown, the dispensing orifice is incorporated into a screw-on base and closed with a small plug molded into the hinged top. The plug and its mating orifice form a satisfactory seal for most viscous pharmaceutical products.

Flip-Top Closures for Solids

Although the flip-top closure was first introduced for liquid products that flow readily through small orifices, the convenience of this closure has now moved into the realm of solid dosage forms. Maalox antacid tablets are now available in a container with a CT polypropylene closure that features a flush hinge flip lid over a very large orifice through which the tablets can be dispensed [2]. The flush hinge design is easier for the consumer to handle and runs better on filling lines than those with protruding hinges. The two-piece feature of flip-top closures allows different colors to be used for the lid and the threaded base. In the Maalox package, different lid colors were chosen to match the flavors of the tablets, but other packaging purposes can be achieved by this color flexibility.

Closures with Applicators

The traditional iodine bottle closure and containers fitted with droppers may be the most familiar pharmaceutical examples of applicator-type closures. In addition to rods or droppers, this closure type may feature brushes — for cosmetics and adhesives — or daubers, which are felt or cotton pads affixed to a rod. Glass or plastic droppers can be calibrated for the dispensing of precise dosages.

Fitment Closures

This term is used for closure designs which regulate the flow of liquids or solids out of the container. They may be inserted into the neck of the container, which is then separately capped, or incorporated directly into the closure itself. Dropper tips are used with squeeze bottles to allow the dispensing of one drop at a time. Sifter and shaker designs contain holes through which powders and granules can be shaken or poured. These can contain a variety of hole sizes and are often closed with a revolving disc. The variety of designs available is almost as large as the variety of products they enclose.

Spray and Pump Dispensers

Sprayers displace a fixed volume of fluid when a piston is depressed inside an accumulator. The fluid exits through an orifice which can be designed to produce spray patterns from fine to very coarse. The quantity of fluid dispensed per stroke depends on the viscosity of the fluid. For example, common spray and pump dispensers deliver from 0.5 to 1 cc of water per stroke. All the common plastics (HDPE, PVC, PP) are used to fabricate these closure types.

To make pump dispensers easy to use by the elderly, some are now designed so that the entire container can be squeezed. This makes it simpler for those with limited hand strength to access the product without depending on only one digit to depress a pump.

Single Dose Dispensers

Increasingly, closures are being asked to dispense precise single dose quantities of medication and to thwart efforts by children to get more than one dose out of the container. One example, shown in Figure 6.11, uses a lock and key mechanism which is set by the pharmacist to produce the proper dose [3]. This mechanism positions the piston in the variable-volume measuring chamber. After the patient aligns the measuring chamber with the exit spout, inversion of the container releases the required dosage.

Another precise-dispensing design (Figure 6.12) takes a cubic centimeter of product and divides it into drops for exact dosing. When the container is inverted, the product dispenses automatically without shaking or squeezing. A variety of orifice sizes are provided to allow for viscosity and surface tension differences [4].

Closures and Compliance

The increasing problem with compliance that is discussed elsewhere in this book has been tackled by closure designers as well.

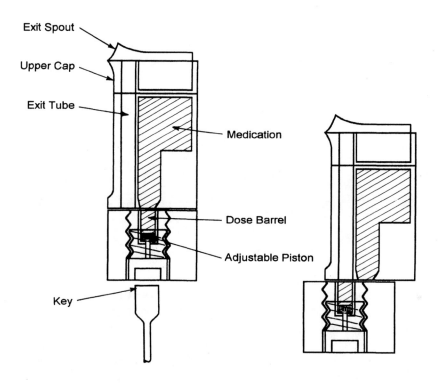

(a) Dose barrel aligned with medication chamber

(b) Dose barrel aligned with exit tube and spout

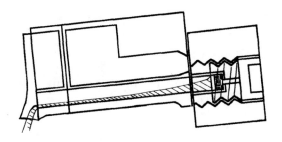

(c) Container inverted, dose dispensed

FIGURE 6.11. Preset single dose dispenser.

193

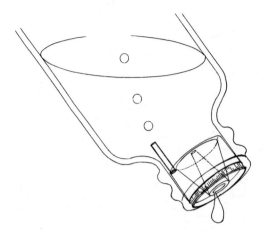

FIGURE 6.12. Precise-dispensing closure.

One has come up with a fitment that is adhered to the top of a closure with two-sided tape. It counts the number of times a closure has been opened and displays the result in a window. Different models are used for different dosage regimens which can range from one dose per day to four. Another operates by advancing each time the closure is removed but then displays through a window the day when the next dosage is to be taken. This one includes a tamper evident feature: before the closure is first removed, a green panel shows through the window. This panel turns to red when the closure is first removed [5].

Closure Materials

Plastics

Thermoplastics are the most widely used materials for drug packaging closures. Four plastic types are most commonly used.

Polypropylene

The excellent stress-crack resistance of PP makes it the plastic of choice for hinged closures. PP has the best heat resistance (sterilizability) of any of the common polyolefins and also has good resistance to solvents, acids, alkalis, oils and greases. It is relatively rigid, which is usually an advantage, and is easy to emboss. Its relatively high strength allows the use of thin flexible sections. Additional rigidity can be achieved by using various mineral fillers as reinforcing materials.

Low Density Polyethylene

LDPE is inferior to PP or HDPE except in flexibility and resiliency. Since it is the lowest cost plastic, it is sometimes used when its inferior properties are not a drawback.

High Density Polyethylene

Like PP, HDPE is stiff and hard but has inferior stress-crack resistance, particularly in the presence of some solvents. It also tends to warp and lose torque, but has better gas barrier characteristics than LDPE. In cost it lies between LDPE and PP, so it is used in situations that demand performance better than LDPE but not as good as the higher cost PP.

Polystyrene

Rubber-modified polystyrene has adequate ductility and rigidity for closure use but its poor gas barrier and thermal resistance make it a mediocre closure candidate as compared to the other thermoplastic alternatives.

Thermosets

Thermosetting phenolic and urea-formaldehyde compositions are rigid, dense, and have good elevated temperature capability. Their excellent dimensional stability ensures minimum slippage over threads, but if overtightened, they may crack. Their use today is largely traditional, since the better fabrication flexibility, lower cost and linerless capability of the thermoplastics make them increasingly popular, particularly for complex designs.

Metal

Although largely displaced by plastics, metal closures are still used to some extent by U.S. drug companies, more commonly on glass than on plastic containers. Aluminum continues to be used

for roll-on closures and for elastomer overcaps on vials for injectables. Steel closures are rarely used for drugs, except in aerosol
cans.

Elastomers

The use of these unique materials for vial closures is discussed
in detail above and in Chapter Four.

Joining the Closure to the Container

Separate closures are joined to the container by a sequence of
operations. These begin with the charging of the closures to a
bulk hopper from which they are sorted and aligned by vibratory
or rotary motion and fed to a capping device. In this device, the
closure is picked up and applied to the container using rotary motion for CT types and downward pressure for snap-on types. The
rotary motion can be applied to the cap or to the container, and
can be intermittent or as fast as 2000 caps per minute on continuous high speed machines. As noted above, the application
torque must be measured and controlled to ensure the proper
seal. Marring of the cap must be avoided during the later stages of
tightening, either by matching the interior finish of the tightening
chuck to the finish of the cap or by lining the chuck jaws with a
high friction rubber doughnut. As might be expected, a wide variety of machine types are available to perform these various operations [6].

CLOSURE LINERS

A closure liner, also called a *wad*, is any structure, usually
resilient, that is manufactured separately and inserted into the
closure to make a seal between the closure and the container on
which it fits.

These devices serve four basic sealing functions:

- to provide a tight seal between the closure and the
  container
- to provide a barrier against loss of volatile components of
  the product being packaged or against ingress of
  atmospheric gases such as oxygen or water vapor

- to prevent loss of liquid contents if the container is turned upside down
- to prevent any undesirable interaction between the package contents and the closure

Closure liners must not be confused with innerseals described below under tamper evidence. Innerseals are applied to the bottle lip in various ways and serve to indicate tampering and to seal the container, although closure liners, being permanent, perform the latter function more effectively.

For a closure liner to successfully perform the four functions listed above, it must resist attack by the contents of the package, it must not interact with the contents in a way that would alter their efficacy, potency or safety, it must be compatible with whatever sterilization method is used for the package and it must release cleanly when the closure is removed.

Structure and Materials

Traditional closure liners consist of two basic components, a backing and a facing. The backing contributes sufficient compressability and resilience for a tight seal. The facing provides gas barrier and isolates the closure from the package contents.

A wide variety of materials and material combinations are available for closure liners. Thus it is difficult to generalize in a summary fashion about liner constructions. However, most backings are made either of pulpboard, chipboard, cork agglomerate, feltboard, rubber, plastic or newsprint plus various waxes and adhesives. Most facings fall into six categories:

- coated paper
- paper laminations
- unsupported foil
- coated foil
- film/foil laminations
- plastic film

Each of these major categories has numerous subcategories. For example, paper laminations include paper/foil, paper/PET, paper/foil/PVC, paper/PVDC, paper/foil/PE, and so forth. Coated foil can be foil coated with PE, PVC, PVDC, PP, ionomer or EAA.

Traditional structures consisting of a backing adhered to a facing are giving way to lower cost, all-plastic liner compositions. These structures, made of PE or PP, can be either solid monolayers or multilayer coextrusions. The latter frequently consist of a foam core with solid plastic layers on top and bottom. They can be combined with facing materials such as foil if the plastic alone cannot perform all the required functions, but the versatility of plastics makes such combinations usually unnecessary; foil is now found mainly performing the tamper evident function as an induction-sealed innerlayer rather than as a component of the liner itself.

An alternative approach is the use of flowed-in compounds rather than a separately made disc-shaped liner. These compounds are variously plastisols, organisols, or latices applied and then heated to drive off the solvent. While these compounds generally provide good seals, they have some drawbacks: solvent must be driven off and residual solvent may remain to contaminate the package contents.

Closure liners became necessary adjuncts of the closure system in the days when caps were made of either metal or thermosetting plastics—both hard materials which could not readily be deformed by application torque to closely fit the bottle or jar lip and create a tight seal. Although they are still used in conjunction with the softer, flexible thermoplastic polyolefins, cap designers are using the fabrication flexibility of thermoplastics to create linerless caps which have built in features that produce a sufficiently tight seal for most drugs.

The seal of a linerless closure is achieved by a variety of molded embossments that form diaphragms, plugs, valve seats, deflecting membranes or rings, all of which press upon or grasp the bead of the container finish.

CHILD-RESISTANT CLOSURES

Child-resistant (CR) closures or packaging are those which defy penetration by young children but can be opened by adults. Although this kind of packaging can be traced back to the 19th century, Congressional interest in such packages began in 1966 and led to the establishment of protocols for CR packages. The years that followed saw a steady increase in the number of CR closures used in pharmaceutical packaging. The Department of

Commerce estimates that today, about 70% of the roughly seven billion drug package closures are designed to be child resistant.

The Poison-Prevention Packaging Act and Its Provisions

In late 1970, Congress passed the U.S. Poison-Prevention Packaging Act and placed enforcement first under the FDA and then in 1973 under the newly formed Consumer Product Safety Commission (CPSC). As time passed, more substances were added to the list of those falling under the regulations. Table 6.1 shows the entire current list with the exception of household pesticides which are regulated by the EPA rather than the CPSC or the FDA [7]. The data in the table indicate the effectiveness of the Act by showing the decrease in ingestions of each substance by children under five since each became regulated [8]. Although these data are now old, with 1982 the latest year, they nevertheless clearly show the beneficial effect of the Act. The data for aspirin, which prior to the Act was the leading cause of childhood poisoning deaths, are particularly encouraging [9].

The significance of these decline figures is better appreciated when we note that there were 8146 accidental aspirin ingestions

Table 6.1. CRC regulated substances and ingestion history.

Regulated Substance	Effective Year	Ingestion % Decrease Since Effective Year
Aspirin	1972	78
Controlled Drugs	1972	70
Methyl Salicylate	1972	70
Furniture Polish	1972	67
Fire Starters	1973	74
Turpentine	1973	86
Lye Preparations	1973	86
Sulfuric Acid	1973	insufficient data
Methanol	1973	insufficient data
Oral Prescription Drugs	1974	46
Ethylene Glycol	1974	57
Iron Preparations	1977	55
Paint Solvents	1977	72
Acetaminophen	1980	26

in 1972, resulting in forty-six deaths [10]. By 1982, the number had dropped to 1753 and prescription drugs took over as the most frequently accidentally ingested drug.

The prominence of aspirin in the early statistics was well known prior to the passage of the Act. In fact, the two largest baby aspirin manufacturers had converted to a safety closure by 1970, although conversion of adult aspirin containers did not generally take place until after the regulations took effect [11].

The regulations for each of the drug categories listed in Table 6.1 are quite detailed and contain a few specific exemptions. For details on limitations and exemptions, the reader should consult the applicable 16 CFR sections [12].

In an attempt to reconcile the conflicting needs of the infirm with children's need for protection, the regulations provide that a customer or prescriber can request a non-child-resistant closure, but prohibit the pharmacist from making this choice for the customer. In addition, except for substances dispensed directly by physicians or dentists, the packager may put a regulated substance in one package size that does not meet the regulations if he also supplies that substance in packages that do. The non-complying packages must bear a label stating, "This package for households without young children" [13].

If the drug is dispensed by a pharmacist without repackaging, both he and the manufacturer are responsible for seeing that the closure is child resistant. If the drug is repackaged by the pharmacist, then he is responsible [14]. Many prescription drugs are packaged by the manufacturer in containers that do not go directly to the ultimate consumer; bottles containing 500 tablets are an example. In such cases, child-resistant closures (CRCs) are not required.

Prescription drugs that are intended for topical application to the teeth or for administration by inhalation are not required to have CRCs — only orally ingested prescription drugs are regulated [15].

Test Procedures

The original regulations specify in great detail the procedures that must be used to determine whether a particular closure design meets the requirements [16]. In summary, the package is evaluated by a panel consisting of 200 healthy children between the ages of forty-two months and fifty-one months and 100 normal adults, eighteen to forty-five years old and 70% female. The adult age range was chosen to fit what the Commission believed was the age range and sex distribution to which most children under five were exposed.

The children are asked to open a package and are given five minutes to do so. If they fail, they are shown how, told they can use their teeth, and given another five minutes. The package passes if at least 85% of the children fail in the first five minutes and 80% in the second five. Adults are allowed five minutes to open and reclose the package without any coaching. The system passes if at least 90% of the adults are successful.

A blister package fails if more than eight blisters are opened by the children in five minutes or if they have opened enough blisters to gain access to a dose that would cause bodily harm to a 25-pound child or if at least one blister has not been opened by at least 90% of the adults. Interestingly, testers find that rather than getting bored after penetrating one blister, many children will keep opening them until the time elapses. On the average, children will open between three and five blisters in the time allotted. By so doing, they often get at enough pills to acquire a toxic dose. For example, 1 gram is a toxic dose of acetaminophen for a 25-pound child — the normal acetaminophen tablet contains 500 mg.

Thus, although there are many reasons for blisters to be increasingly used to package drugs, a major drawback is that for products where a child-toxic dose consists of a few (1–3) units, it is hard to design a child-safe blister that can also be penetrated by 90% of adults in five minutes [17]. Nevertheless, at least one such design has appeared. It is used for Children's Tylenol (McNeilab Inc.) in the form of 160 mg caplets and also for capsules containing Richardson-Vicks' NyQuil liquid cold medicine. The design consists of a 5" × 2" card, perforated along its long axis, with the transparent side made of PET film and the opaque side of paperboard — a combination that resists "push-through" access. To open a blister, the card must first be torn in half along the perforation and then torn in a direction perpendicular to the perforation beginning at a notch. The second tear releases the caplet. This package successfully passes the child panel test because it is difficult for young children to learn a process that requires two separate, sequential motions; in this case the two tear steps which must be performed in sequence [18]. Unfortunately, this design may be marginal in ease of adult access—the NyQuil graphics include the comment, "If it [the package] is difficult to open, use scissors"!

Child-Resistant Closure Designs

Four major assumptions about children aged forty-two to fifty-one months underlie the design of successful CRCs:

- They cannot readily perform two different motions at the same time.
- They can neither read nor determine alignments but can learn quickly by watching adults.
- They are not strong but are likely to be more persistent and will use tools such as table edges or teeth to help themselves.
- Their teeth and fingernails are sharp and can slide under and into gaps.

The three most common reclosable CR closure types are the press-turn, squeeze-turn, and combination lock. Press-turn involves the simultaneous application of downward pressure while unscrewing the cap. Squeeze-turn uses a freely rotating soft plastic overcap which engages an inner threaded cap or disengages a locking mechanism when pressure is applied to the sidewall. Combination lock caps use components which must be correctly oriented before the cap can be removed. The most common embodiment is the snap-off cap which can be removed only if an arrow on the cap is aligned with a matching arrow on the bottle lip. The thread on the bottle lip is interrupted at the arrow. A protrusion on the cap fits under the thread on the bottle lip and prevents opening unless it is aligned with the interruption in the thread.

A variant related to the press-turn closure is sometimes used for all-plastic containers. It consists of a bottle neck which is threaded at the top and then, after a straight cylindrical section, has two projecting rings at the bottom. The lower ring is larger than the upper and equipped with a molded-in tab and a hook. When the cap is screwed on by means of the upper threads, a recessed section at the cap bottom, which extends partway around the cap and is interrupted by small vertical baffles, fits over the hook on the tab. As rotation is continued, the hook is depressed by one of the small vertical baffles and is then released as rotation carries it past this baffle. This produces an audible *click*, but more importantly, prevents unscrewing of the cap unless the tab is pushed down until the hook can clear the baffle.

For the rare situations where aerosol cans contain CR-regulated products, a cap is available which must be pried up with a coin or tool [19]. After dispensing, the cap can be reinstalled in a CR configuration.

Most CR designs require two hands to open the closure. At least one design is available, however, which allows a hinged top to pop up when pressure is applied to both sides of the container [20].

In the nonreclosable category, both blister packages and sealed pouches can be child-resistant. So far, few blister designs meet both the child-resistant panel tests and the easy-opening requirements of the elderly. As noted above, the blister package that is used for Children's Tylenol and NyQuil meets both requirements. Plastic pouches are rarely used for drugs, particularly those of the prescription variety. To be CR, a pouch construction would need to be unusually strong to resist the teeth of a determined four-year-old, even though hard-to-open plastic bags are a source of irritation to adult consumers nationwide.

Other special package designs such as aerosol cans and pump sprays are regarded by the CPSC as appropriate CR candidates, but are infrequently used for prescription drugs.

Recent Developments

As time passed, it became apparent that CR packages were causing problems in the older segment of the population. Increasingly, this led to the deliberate purchase of drugs in non-CR packages or to leaving the CR closure off the package. A CPSC study [21] in 1989 of accidental ingestion of medication by children under five showed that:

- Of the medications that were prescriptions, 44% were not in CR packages.
- Forty percent of the medications (prescription or not) were not originally packaged in CR containers.
- Seventeen percent of those medications ingested by children were in containers that were not properly

resecured prior to ingestion. In these cases, either the drug was out of the container entirely, the top was left open, or a new top had been put on the container.

Reacting to these results, CPSC has proposed to substitute a panel of adults aged sixty to seventy-five for the younger adult panel heretofore used [22]. The time allowed for adult opening and resecuring would be reduced to one minute, since the Commission now feels that a five-minute period greatly exceeds the time that consumers would be willing to spend opening any package. The one-minute period would be preceded by a period of thirty seconds that the adult could use to become familiar with how the package operates. If it is found by experience that for some reason it is not feasible to make this panel age substitution, the Commission will reduce the opening time by the younger panel to thirty seconds after a thirty-second familiarization period. Other changes of a largely statistical nature are also proposed to reduce testing costs, plus a test by children to determine if the package has been properly resecured by the adults. These changes, while benefitting older people, are being proposed principally to give greater protection to children who are still vulnerable to CR packages that are not handled properly by older people, who by the year 2030 are expected to make up 25% of the population [23].

The substitution of an older panel for a younger one worries packagers who use blister packages because they fear that these package types may fail the test by the older panel [24]. The Healthcare Compliance Packaging Council, through its president, Daniel Gerner, argues that if CPSC-approved blister package designs fail an older panel test, the many compliance and safety advantages of blister packages and their related unit dose capability may be lost. A satisfactory compromise between these two conflicting objectives might be reached if blister packages which do not have a peel-off backing were pronounced CR by the CPSC, since they would pass an older panel test, and the compliance, convenience and safety features of blister packages could be retained [25].

In a recent survey, ease of opening was termed "extremely important" by 82% of consumers over age sixty [26]. The drug packager's response to this need is not yet evident, but a few ideas have surfaced:

- In Europe, a plastic closure is now commercial that has two pairs of molded-in prongs between which the user can insert a knife or similar tool to use as a lever. Although available in the U.S., it has not yet found application here.
- Variations on this tool-assisted closure concept have been proposed [27]. Two involve an outer cap–inner cap scheme like the basic push-and-turn design but with a provision for inserting a tool such as a key or a pencil. The tool locks the two caps together and provides ample leverage so that the inner cap can be turned off without squeezing or pushing down on the outer cap.
- Naldecon Senior DX cough syrup from Bristol Laboratories is packaged in a square glass bottle with a knurled cap and accompanied by directions for opening printed in type three times larger than customary [28].

Although most OTC drugs are not required to have CRCs, drug packagers are increasingly using CR designs on their OTC products. One recent British journal states categorically that "most over-the-counter medicines are now packed in child-resistant opaque bottles" [29]. We believe this to be true for the U.S. as well, since the U.S. has historically led the world in the use of CR packages.

As for drug package closures generally, the design freedom offered by plastics has been the major factor in the increasing dominance of plastic, as compared to metal, in CR closures. The Bureau of Census reports that in 1986, over 75% of CRC closures for regulated products were plastic [30]. There is little doubt that newer data would show an even greater preponderance of plastic CR closures.

TAMPER EVIDENCE

In October 1982, seven people in the Chicago area died after ingesting Tylenol capsules that had been laced with cyanide.

This tragedy set in motion activity by government and industry which still continues: manufacturers try to create packages which will prevent such incidents and government continues to update regulations as new tamper evident technology is developed.

The immediate reaction by Johnson & Johnson, the manufacturer of Tylenol, was to temporarily withdraw the product while they incorporated three new features in the package: a seal glued across the neck of the bottle, a neck band heat shrunk around the cap and neck of the bottle, and glued flaps on the outer box. In addition, warning labels were affixed to the box and to the bottle inside that cautioned users to reject the product if they found any safety seals broken. These package changes reportedly cost J&J two to four cents per package [31].

FDA Regulations for Tamper Evident Packaging

The FDA reacted to the poisonings with equal swiftness. On November 5, 1982, the *Federal Register* contained an announcement of their new rules, now embodied in 21 CFR 211.132, designed to thwart tampering with OTC drug products.

Definitions

They began by defining what they originally called a "tamper resistant" package as follows: "[one which has] an indicator or barrier to entry which, if breached or missing, can reasonably be expected to provide visible evidence to consumers that tampering has occurred" [32]. Later usage improved on this definition by substituting the term "tamper evident," which recognizes that the present tamper evident package designs can at best only provide evidence that tampering has occurred. They will not discourage or foil the sophisticated tamperer who has specialized tools available.

Regulations

- The tamper evidence indicator or barrier must either be distinctive by design, such as an aerosol container, or be an identifying characteristic (pattern, name, logo) that makes the package difficult to duplicate.
- Each package must bear a prominent statement that alerts the consumer to the tamper evident feature it incorporates. This statement must be so located that it will be unaffected if the tamper evident feature is breached or missing.

- The products covered by the regulations are:
  - all OTC drug products: nasal, otic, ophthalmic, rectal, vaginal, and oral, except for insulin, dentifrices, and topical dermatological products
  - oral cosmetic liquids such as mouthwashes, gargles, and breath fresheners
  - contact lens solutions and tablets

Later exemptions added were lozenges, ammonia inhalant ampules, aerosol products and compressed medical oxygen.

Breadth of Applicability

The FDA's original intent was to regulate products accessible to the public on store shelves. Products not accessible to the public in this way are exempt from the regulations. These would be, for example:

- products sold directly to a hospital, an institution or a physician
- products sold in vending machines
- products sold through the mail or door-to-door

Acceptable Package Forms

As part of the regulations, the FDA gave examples of acceptable package forms or technologies, keeping the wording general to encourage innovation and to give packagers as much freedom as possible. The original list, which was clearly indicated to be just a beginning with the expectation that it would change, contained eleven different forms [33]:

1. *Film wrappers.* A transparent film imprinted with a distinctive design is wrapped securely around the container in such a way that it must be cut or torn to get at the product. The wrapper must have some identifying characteristic that cannot be readily duplicated, such as a pattern, name, picture, or logo. Simply tinting the wrapper is not adequate.

   The wrapper must fit tightly, as does a shrink wrapped film. A tear strip is helpful, not only for ease of opening, but also because it is extremely difficult to replace without specialized equipment. A film with overlapping sealed end flaps is not adequate unless the manufacturer is sure the ends cannot be opened without leaving some evidence of the breach. That can be a very difficult requirement for the conventional glued overwrap to meet.

2. *Blister or strip packs.* These are dosage units individually sealed in plastic/foil/paper constructions. It must be necessary to tear the compartment to get at the product, and the backing materials must not be separable from the blister without leaving evidence that that has happened. For obvious reasons, push-through backings are better than backings which peel off.

3. *Bubble packs.* These resemble #2 except that the plastic bubble surrounding the product is mounted on a card. The comments listed under #2 also apply to this category.

4. *Heat shrunk bands or wrappers.* These are bands or wrappers with a distinctive design that are shrunk around the neck and closure to seal the union between them. The seal must be torn to release the closure. This approach works best if the band is made wide enough to extend well down the sides of the container. Cellulose-based wet shrink seals are not acceptable, since many people know how to remove these nondestructively by soaking them in water.

5. *Foil, paper, or plastic pouches.* Such pouches must be torn to get at the product and must feature a distinctive design. The end seals, if breached, must show evidence of entry.

6. *Bottle mouth inner seals.* These are materials such as paper, foil, plastic films, plastic foams, or combinations thereof, with a distinctive design, sealed to the mouth of the container under the closure. They must be torn to get at the product. There are three common types:
   - A glassine film with a wax-coated pulp backing. Adhesive on the glassine holds it fast to the bottle finish when the cap and its pulp liner are removed. The cap liner facilitates resealing after the glassine membrane is removed.
   - Foamed polystyrene discs that have a pressure-sensitive adhesive to adhere the innerseal to the bottle finish.
   - Induction-sealed innerseals: these may be either:
     — adhesive or plastic-coated foil temporarily adhered

with wax to a separating base material, usually a pulp liner, or

- − adhesive or plastic-coated foil permanently glued to chipboard, or
- − adhesive or plastic-coated unsupported foil

The application of an external magnetic field to these structures generates eddy currents in the foil layer. These create enough heat in the foil to melt the plastic or activate the adhesive which then adheres the foil to the finish. In the first type, the heat also melts the wax so the pulp liner can be separated from the innerseal [34].

This method is becoming increasingly popular, since induction sealing is a clean system providing a bond that is quite difficult for a tamperer to penetrate. A widely used structure is a 0.2 mil LDPE adhesive film layer bonded to 1 mil aluminum foil which in turn is wax-bonded to 13 mil pulpboard. Heat generated in the foil layer fuses the LDPE to the bottle lip while simultaneously melting the wax layer to release the pulpboard liner from the foil which is left in place as the closure liner [35].

The presence of an induction-sealed innerseal can be verified by inspection on the filling line. An infrared sensor monitors the temperature in the air space directly above the seal and compares it to the temperature at the side of the bottle. A differential of several degrees, independent of the ambient temperature, will exist if the induction seal has been satisfactorily made.

Foil-based innerseals are often found on semi-bulk containers that are shipped to pharmacists even though such containers are exempt from the tamper evidence regulations. In these cases, the innerseal serves as a moisture barrier. Innerseals and shrink bands are now the most frequently used tamper evident systems.

7. *Tape seals.* These are made of paper or foil and sealed over all carton flaps or a bottle cap with some feature that shows when they have been removed and reapplied.

8. *Breakable cap-ring systems.* These are threaded caps with perforations forming a break line along a band on the lower part of the closure skirt. The band is locked to the container

210   CLOSURES FOR PHARMACEUTICAL PACKAGES

finish by crimping or ratchets. When the closure is twisted off, the band separates from it and remains on the bottle.

The breakaway cap can be installed in place of a conventional cap with little retrofit investment. It is highly visible, well-known to consumers, and quite durable in distribution. Nevertheless, it is not terribly difficult to replace the cap and carefully align it with the broken ring in such a way that most consumers would not notice that the joints between cap and ring had been broken. The effectiveness of this approach is enhanced if the original breaking action makes a clearly audible noise.

The tearaway band is a variant of the breakaway cap that employs an LDPE band that must be completely removed before the cap can be taken off. A protruding tab is usually provided to facilitate the tear. Many nonthreaded tamper evident closures use this approach, although it is easier for a tamperer to foil than the breakaway cap, and offers less obvious evidence of tampering.

9. *Sealed tubes or plastic blind-end heat sealed tubes.* Both ends of a tube are sealed and must be punctured to obtain product. A crimped end tube is acceptable so long as the crimped end cannot be breached and then refolded without leaving signs that this has occurred. In practice, this means that the crimped end must be heat sealed.

10. *Sealed cartons.* The official comment on sealed cartons is "All flaps of a carton are securely sealed and the carton must be visibly damaged when opened to remove the product" [36]. However, the FDA's position as of early 1988 was that cartons sealed by glueing the end flaps are an "unacceptable technology" and hence not in compliance.

11. *Aerosol containers.* The FDA regards aerosol containers as being "inherently tamper resistant" by design, but they recommend direct printing of the label on the container to prevent label substitution.

12. *All-metal and composite cans.* This category was added to the list in 1987. It did not appear on the original list because cans were then rarely used for OTC drugs. Later growth in use of these container types stimulated their addition. To meet the requirements, the tops and bottoms of composite cans must be joined to the can body in such a way that they

cannot be removed without visible damage. Direct printing of the label on the can is recommended.

Ease of Opening

At the outset, the FDA and packagers recognized that the inclusion of tamper evident features would make packages more difficult to open, a problem which might be serious for elderly consumers. Both the FDA and the CPSC studied this problem and concluded that although added difficulties existed, they did not warrant adding a standard of tamper evident package access [37]. However, their position is that the needs of the elderly and infirm must be kept in mind and that ideally, a tamper evident feature should be "delicate, fragile, and simple by design" to enhance easy openability [38].

The two agencies also made it clear that tamper evident packaging does not change in any way the status of the regulations for CRCs, or the reverse; in other words, there is no connection between the two needs.

The conclusion reached by the FDA and the CPSC in this study will probably be altered as the population continues to age and the needs of the elderly and infirm are increasingly brought to the attention of packagers. Certainly most tamper evident designs make life more difficult for older people, and we can expect evolution towards designs which are more user-friendly for the elderly. In this connection, plastic closures and devices have been found to be easier for the elderly to open, a fact that will continue the trend towards plastics and away from metal. A good example of this approach is a PP closure which incorporates a tamper evident tear ring along with a flip-top cap which makes frequent re-entry much simpler [39].

Capsule Problems

In 1986, three people died after ingesting cyanide-laced capsules of Extra Strength Excedrin. The manufacturer, Bristol-Myers, reacted in part by discontinuing their use of capsules for this product and other manufacturers also began to move away from capsules [40]. Those who stayed with capsules began to seal the joint between the two capsule halves in various ways [41]. For this purpose, the FDA approved the use of sonic welding, gelatin banding, or sealing thermally or with solvents, but warned, "The use of an acceptable capsule sealing technology will enhance the tamper resistant features already utilized for the product's packaging but will not be considered as a substitute for the required tamper resistant feature" [42]. The FDA later went even further, requiring packagers that used unsealed capsules to incorporate two tamper evident features in their packages, one of which could be eliminated if sealed capsules were used [43].

Shrink Wrapping vs. Shrink Bands

Manufacturers of clear plastic shrink films moved quickly after the first Tylenol incident to point out to packagers the many inherent and effective tamper evident features of their product, buttressing their arguments with the results of a public opinion survey which showed that 90% of the respondents favored shrink wrap over glued cartons and 75% preferred shrink wrap to shrink bands. As a result, some drug companies adopted a shrink wrap over the entire drug container [44]. As time passed, however, the lower cost and greater simplicity of shrink neck bands led to the more frequent use of this latter approach, even though overall shrink wrap is harder to unobtrusively penetrate than is a shrink neck band.

Shrink wrap is still used, particularly when it can be used to perform other functions such as the co-packaging of a device along with the drug container. A good example is the recent introduction of a flu medication in a PET bottle accompanied by a dosage cup placed over the primary closure and securely affixed to the package by shrink wrapping the entire assembly [45].

Some users of the shrink wrap approach have upgraded their security by marking the shrink wrap on line with an ink-jet coder, rather than relying on preprinted film, feeling that this approach makes duplication of the film by a tamperer more difficult [46].

One problem with shrink wrapping is that if it is removed by a tamperer, it may not be missed, even though the container label warns that it should be present. Shrink bands, which should have the same drawback, have become so pervasive that they are more likely to be missed.

Skin packaging is a technique closely related to shrink packaging and would appear to be an even more attractive approach since a skin package is almost invisible, yet tightly retains the contents [47]. To date, no drug manufacturer has adopted this technique, because early skin packaging films left cloudy areas on the wrapped array, a phenomenon that skin packagers refer to as "the wet look." This problem has recently been overcome and some manufacturers may adopt this technique in the future, although it would suffer the same drawback as shrink wrapping [48].

Conversion to Tamper Evident Packaging

The addition of tamper-evidence features to existing packages was not a simple process for packagers. Manufacturers now converting prescription drugs to OTC products have the same set of problems: additional capital investment and the need to shoehorn facilities into already crowded buildings. This factor is more severe for some approaches than others. For example, conversion of a simple closure to a breakaway cap may not involve these problems and is one reason for the adoption of this tamper evident option in preference to shrink wrap, shrink bands, or innerseal membranes. Line efficiencies are adversely affected by the additional step, materials costs increase, and engineering time is needed to design and shepherd the adoption of a new package. This array of problems and others is well covered in a recent article which describes Pfizer's introduction of their first OTC oral liquid [49]. In their case, a CRC was also required, further complicating the problem.

Recent Developments

In 1991, two residents of the state of Washington died after consuming Sudafed capsules contaminated with cyanide. The capsules were sealed with a blue gelatin band, blister packaged with a printed backing, and cartoned with the flaps taped closed — more tamper evident features than are required [50]. The tampering was amateurish and obvious: the safety tab on the end flaps had been slit and reglued; the foil backing on the blister pack was pulled back and either not reglued or resecured with tape; the poisoned capsules were different in size and color than the rest, had no blue sealing band, and carried no printing. All this once again shows that lack of consumer awareness is a major factor in the continuing success of evilly motivated tamperers [51].

There was immediate speculation that this third capsule incident might lead to the banning of capsules [50]. David Kessler, the current FDA director, signalled as much on March 7, 1991, as did the Centers for Disease Control [52]. The National Wholesale Drug Manufacturer's Association cites these advantages of capsules to show that eliminating them as a dosage form would be a mistake:

- They are easy to swallow.
- They can be printed for identification purposes.
- They resist shipping damage better than tablets.
- Some medicines cannot be tabletted.
- They do not require inactive ingredients that may upset some consumers.
- They offer an excellent way to provide timed release.
- Many customers prefer them.

Kessler also voiced the opinion widely held amongst manufacturers and trade associations that, "Consumers must maintain their vigilance. They must look twice before taking any OTC product" [53]. This point is an important one: if consumers are not vigilant, no amount of technology (with the possible exception of packaging every OTC product in a metal can) will prevent the recurrence of these unfortunate incidents.

Although a 1983 University of Michigan study showed that most consumers could not distinguish tampered from untampered packages in nine out of eleven examples where approved tamper evident features were present, more recent data shows that the percentage of consumers who avoided buying a product because it appeared to have been tampered with rose from 31% in 1987 to over 50% in 1989 [54]. Even so, parallel studies also show that over 50% of consumers are "generally indifferent" to tampering and to tamper evident features on packages [55].

One unobvious motive for tampering with drugs was brought to light in 1986 by an interview [56] with an unsuccessful drug tamperer who had been apprehended. His motives were strictly financial: he tampered with a capsuled product and then notified the company, in the hopes of generating enough publicity to affect the price of the company's stock which he had recently sold short! This anecdote reinforces the argument that tampering will always be with us, that there are no practical, inexpensive tamper *proof* solutions, and that consumer vigilance is a vital ingredient in the preventive mix.

Some engineers skilled in this area go further: they believe that the best tamper evident devices are effective only against *in-store* tampering. One has stated that his experts can unobtrusively tamper with any tamper evident system if they can remove the package from the store and use specialized techniques [57].

New Approaches to Tamper Evidence

The persistence of tampering and the desire of drug companies to upgrade their designs, reduce their costs, and make tamper evident packages more user-friendly all guarantee that this facet of drug packaging will continue to consume the energy of drug packaging designers and engineers. Noted here are some new approaches to this problem that illustrate the variety of activities underway.

A significant improvement on the glued flap box has been introduced by Rexham. It consists of a standard folding carton whose ends, if breached, show the word "opened" in a polyester film window. Resealing the carton will not obliterate the word. Adoption of this approach is easy if the manufacturer already has cartoning equipment. Rexham's market research revealed a preference for this tamper evidence approach, as opposed to overwraps, shrink bands, and tape seals, from the standpoint of both tamper evidence and easy openability [58].

Some effort is devoted to schemes which cause some highly visible irreversible change in package appearance:

- Packages may include materials that change color when exposed to air.
- Package materials may change color when ripped.
- Optical fibers in bottle caps might collect room light and cause a window to shine unless the bottle is opened, destroying the fiber integrity.
- Multilayered plastic films having extremely thin layers of various inorganic materials vacuum deposited thereon change color and/or appearance depending on viewing angle, but when they are ripped open, this characteristic disappears [59].

- Safety buttons that pop up when the container is opened allowing air to replace the vacuum inside are now used on baby food jars and have the advantage that purchasers of that product are familiar with the feature.
- Pressure sensitive holograms in the form of 2 mil films, if used as tapes, will break apart into a distinctive checkerboard design which could signal removal. Closely related is a frangible PVC pressure sensitive hologram that, after application, cannot be removed in one piece but breaks up into many pieces if removal is attempted [60].
- Threaded bottle closures which, when rotated to open, tear a membrane to reveal a characteristic color under a transparent overcap.
- Capsules may be double coated with a material which hardens after coating and obviously fractures if anyone attempts to breach the capsule [60].

One of several new requirements being considered by the FDA is an improvement in labeling. The new approach would include:

- standardization of the language that announces the tamper evident features of the package
- graphic enhancement (color contrast, clear separation from other label printing, larger type size, etc.) of the tamper evident portion of the message
- requiring the labeling statement to be carried on surfaces other than caps and package inserts

The FDA may also require the label to indicate that unsealed capsules are in the package and tamper evident features be more consistent among the various package sizes used for a product line [62].

Many tamper evident packages have relied on an extra layer of protection: a total overwrap, a neck band, a carton which might not otherwise be needed, etc. These may now run afoul of recent consumer sentiment against over-packaging and tilt future choices toward solutions such as breakaway caps, innerseals, or blister packages, although the latter may also be viewed as over-packaging compared to a plastic bottle.

REFERENCES

1. "Teflon" is a registered trademark of E. I. du Pont de Nemours & Co., Inc.
2. Anon. 1989. *Food & Drug Packaging* (March):3; Anon. 1990. *J. Packaging Technology* (January):7.
3. Anon. 1989. *Food & Drug Packaging* (July):8.
4. Anon. 1991. *Food & Drug Packaging* (July):30.
5. Ibid., p. 27.
6. Kelsey, R. J. 1988. *Food & Drug Packaging* (May):10.
7. Bakker, M., ed. 1986. *The Wiley Encyclopedia of Packaging Technology.* New York, NY: John Wiley & Sons, p. 167.
8. Ibid.
9. Anon. 1988. *Am. J. Hosp. Pharm.,* 45(Jan.):32.
10. Clarke, A. and W. W. Walton. 1979. *Pediatrics,* 63(5/May):690.
11. Ibid., p. 692.
12. FDA. Title 16 of Code of Federal Regulations (CFR), 1700.1(b)(4), 1700.3, 1700.14, 1700.15, 1700.20.
13. 1990. *Federal Register,* 55(194/Oct. 5):40857.
14. Strauss, S. 1983. *U.S. Pharmacist* (September):34.
15. Ibid., p. 35.
16. FDA. Title 16 of Code of Federal Regulations (CFR), 1700; CPSC Regulations, U.S. Consumer Product Safety Commission, Washington, D.C.
17. Dr. Alexander Perrett, president, Perrett Laboratories, private communication, 1992.
18. Laurence Edzenga, SmithKline Beecham, Inc., private communication, 1992.
19. Anon. 1991. *Food & Drug Packaging* (July):24.
20. Ibid, p. 26.
21. *Federal Register,* op. cit., p. 40860.
22. Ibid., p. 40856.
23. Erickson, G. 1990. *Packaging* (November):24.
24. Larson, M. 1991. *Packaging WESTPACK Show Daily* (September):14.
25. Daniel Gerner, president, Health Care Packaging Council, private communication, 1991.

26. Erickson, G., op. cit.

27. Anon. 1988. *Food & Drug Packaging* (May):8.

28. Erickson, G., op. cit., p. 25.

29. Anon. 1989. Manufacturing Chemist, 60(January):28.

30. *Federal Register*, op. cit., p. 40864.

31. Anon. 1982. Drug *Topics* (December 13).

32. FDA. 1990. Title 21 of Code of Federal Regulations (CFR), 211.132.

33. Lampkin, W. J. 1988. *Pharmaceutical Engineering*, 8(Jan.):25.

34. Bakker, M., ed., op. cit., p. 171.

35. Anon. 1986. *Packaging Digest* (August):58.

36. Lampkin, W. J., op. cit.

37. Bakker, M., ed., op. cit., p. 630.

38. Lampkin, W. J., op. cit.

39. Larson, M. 1989. *Packaging* (May):35.

40. Egan, T. 1991. *New York Times* (March 5):6.

41. Anon. 1986. *Packaging* (December):13.

42. Lampkin, W. J., op. cit.

43. Anon. 1988. *Food & Drug Packaging* (July):3.

44. Jolley, C. 1983. *Pharmaceutical Engineering* (September):21.

45. Anon. 1991. *Packaging Digest* (March):44.

46. Larson, M. 1989. *Packaging* (May):36.

47. Osborn, K. R. and W. A. Jenkins. 1992. *Plastic Films: Technology and Packaging Applications.* Lancaster, PA: Technomic Publishing Co., Inc., p. 171.

48. Burton Spottiswoode, E. I. du Pont de Nemours & Co., Inc., private communication, 1991.

49. Suhr, S. E. 1988. *Pharmaceutical Technology* (September):122.

50. Anon. 1991. *Packaging Digest* (April):26; 1991. *Philadelphia Inquirer*, (March 4):11A.

51. Anon. 1991. *Food & Drug Packaging* (April):23.

52. Anon. 1991. *Philadelphia Inquirer* (March 15):15A.

53. Anon. 1991. *Philadelphia Inquirer* (March 7):9A.

54. Larson, M. 1989. *Packaging* (May):36.

55. Ibid., p. 40.

56. Anon. 1986. *Food & Drug Packaging* (December):10.

57. Anon., private communication.

58. Alan Johnston, Rexham Packaging, Inc., private communication, 1991.
59. Arons, R. and H. Stillman. 1987. *Drugs and Clinical Intelligence* (July):46.
60. O'Brien, R. 1991. *Food & Drug Packaging* (September):22.
61. Anon. 1990. *Food & Drug Packaging* (July):15.
62. Lampkin, W. J., op. cit.

CHAPTER SEVEN

Labels and Labeling

Considering all categories of manufactured products, drugs are close to unique in the importance of the role that labeling plays in their distribution and sale. This is because, unlike most other manufactured products, drugs consist of materials whose identity can rarely be ascertained by visual inspection. Thus, unless the identity and the strength are correctly identified on a label which is an integral part of the package, the consequences to the consumer can literally be fatal. Although the literature offers no modern instance of a fatality that can be unambiguously attributed to an adult mistakenly taking a mislabeled drug, the period 1983–1990 has witnessed forty Class I drug recalls by the FDA with eighteen of these attributed to labeling errors [1,2].

Along with these considerations, there is the additional complication that results from the necessity—often a legal necessity—of presenting more information on a drug package label than is the case with other manufactured products. This becomes extremely difficult when bottles are too small to have the printed matter easily legible to all consumers.

Thus label design, manufacture, and application are elements of the drug packaging process which consume an important fraction of the time and thought of drug packaging engineers and other professionals who are involved in labeling.

LEGAL REQUIREMENTS

The serious consequences of mislabeling and labeling errors have led, not surprisingly, to a significant body of regulations by the FDA that apply to drug package labels and the labeling process. We will outline these here, first for prescription drugs and then for drugs sold over the counter.

Prescription Drugs

Just as a new drug and its container must be approved by the FDA, so must the label for that drug, including any significant changes that are made to the label after the drug has been commercialized. The requirements for the information that must be provided via a label or an insert/outsert or both are incredibly voluminous and detailed: fifty-five pages in the Code of Federal Regulations (CFR) are required to convey it all in legal terminology. The following brief summary is only illustrative and must not be used as a reference. Anyone who needs definitive information on this complex subject, including the many exceptions to the general regulations, must consult the CFR [3].

The label must include:

- name and address of the manufacturer, packager or distributor if these are separate organizations
- National Drug Code (NDC) numbers are *requested* (see the following section for discussion of the NDC). This status may be upgraded to mandatory in the future [4]
- statement of active ingredients and their relative potency; if the drug is intended for parenteral administration, all inactive ingredients must be listed
- statement of the quantity and kind of certain listed ingredients whether active or not
- the established names of the drug, both generic and proprietary, and the dosage form
- net quantity of package contents, which will consist of either a numerical count (of tablets or capsules), weight of other forms of solids or semisolids or volume in the case of liquids
- statement of recommended or usual dosage; this information may have to be included on an insert if it gets too voluminous for the label
- a warning if any habit-forming ingredients are present
- a legend that warns that a prescription is required for dispensing

- the route of administration if not oral
- a statement to the pharmacist on the type of container to be used in any repackaging operation
- the expiration date and lot number

To deal with the difficulty of presenting all this information on a small unit dose container, certain categories of information may be omitted and instead appear on the outer package which must also state the number of unit dose containers enclosed therein.

Package inserts, discussed below, also fall under regulatory purview. For prescription drugs, the inserts must provide the following information [5]:

- a summary of the scientific information essential for safe use of the drug presented in an informative but not promotional way
- a *description* section which includes generally the same information that is required for the label plus the pharmacological or therapeutic class of the drug and the chemical name and structural formula of the active ingredient(s)
- a *clinical pharmacology* section that consists of a summary of the human clinical pharmacological actions of the product
- the diseases and conditions the drug is intended to treat, prevent or diagnose
- a *contraindication* section that describes the situations where the drug should not be used
- a warning of any adverse reaction possibilities or safety hazards
- lengthy sections devoted to *precautions, adverse reactions* and *drug abuse and dependence*
- the recommended usual dosage range
- information on available dosage forms, strengths and dosage form units, data on colors or shapes or NDC numbers used for identification, and special handling directions

Beyond this lengthy list of requirements, certain drugs or drug categories have specific labeling requirements. This list includes glandular preparations, estrogenic hormone preparations, drugs containing mineral oil or wintergreen oil, tannic acid and barium enema preparations, isoproterenol inhalation preparations and nine others [6]. The CFR should be consulted for specifics on these exceptions.

Repackaging and Relabeling of Prescription Drugs by Pharmacists and Physicians

When repackaging and relabeling a prescription drug, the retail pharmacist must include, by federal law, his business name and address, the prescription number and the date it was prescribed or filled, the names of the patient and prescriber and the directions for administration provided by the prescriber. State law may additionally require the pharmacist to supply the patient address; the telephone number of the pharmacy; the drug name, strength, and manufacturer's lot or control number; the expiration date, if any and the name of the manufacturer or distributor [7].

Some packagers make the retail pharmacist's job simpler by including the information that is required for the pharmacist on a special section of the label that can be peeled away, leaving either a blank area or a space for applying the pharmacist's label [8].

Hospital pharmacy repackaging operations, particularly those connected with larger hospitals, tend to resemble the packaging operations of drug manufacturers rather than the extemporaneous operations of retail pharmacists. Thus in the case of hospital pharmacies, the CGMP standards and the packaging and labeling standards of the American Society of Hospital Pharmacists (ASHP) apply with particular pertinence [9].

Pharmacists who are expert on medication errors have assembled a set of recommendations for labeling of repackaged stock containers in the hospital pharmacy [10]. Prominent among these recommendations are:

- Labels should indicate the amount of drugs in each dosage unit.
- Expiration date and storage conditions should be clearly indicated.
- Names of all therapeutically active ingredients should be included.
- Forms intended for dilution or reconstitution should carry appropriate directions.

- Labels for large volume sterile solutions should permit visual inspection of container contents.
- Acceptable route(s) of administration should be included for parenteral preparations.
- Drug strengths, volumes, and amounts must be indicated.

Seven additional recommendations complete this comprehensive list.

Since drug manufacturers do not yet supply all drugs in all the unit dose forms desired by hospital pharmacists, the repackaging of bulk drugs in unit dose packages is still an important activity in many hospital pharmacies. The FDA has published guidelines (not requirements) for the material that should be included on labels for unit dose drugs intended for hospital impatient use. These guidelines apply regardless of who does the packaging, of course [11]. This list is a familiar one:

- drug proprietary name
- drug generic name
- quantity of active ingredients
- name of manufacturer
- lot or control number
- expiration date
- the "may-be-habit-forming" warning statement as required

ASHP has supplemented this list with additional recommendations which add to the above list the following items [12]:

- the dosage form, if special or other than oral
- number of tablets and total dose

ASHP does not regard including the proprietary name as important, but it emphasizes, as do other experts, that the generic name and strength should be the most prominent aspects of the label.

Physicians who directly dispense drugs are not bound by the same requirements as are pharmacists who perform the same function. The FDA says, in part, ". . . physicians . . . [are] . . . exempt from strict compliance with the labeling requirements for prescription drugs" [13].

The rationale behind this liberality is apparently the reluctance of the FDA to interfere with the special physician-patient relationship. Some states have taken issue with this and sought to impose some requirements on physicians.

Parenteral Preparations

USP has set up a special set of requirements for labeling of parenteral preparations. In summary, these state that the label must include:

- the name of the preparation
- the percentage content of a drug in a liquid preparation
- the amount of active ingredient of a dry preparation
- the volume of liquid to be added to prepare an injection or suspension
- the route of administration
- statement of storage conditions
- the expiration date
- the name of the manufacturer and a lot number that will provide access to the complete manufacturing history of the preparation

In addition, USP requires that the label and the container be arranged so that the container remains uncovered for its full length or circumference so that the contents may be visually inspected.

Preparations intended for dialysis, hemofiltration or irrigation must bear on the label statements that they are not intended for intravenous injection [14].

Over-the-Counter Drugs

Whereas prescription drug labels for the consumer carry minimal information about the drug itself, the FDA requires that OTC labels be more detailed so that consumers can properly use the products without the advice of a healthcare professional. As a consequence, the label on an OTC drug includes:

1. Name and identity of the product
2. What the product will do, i.e., "antacid," "analgesic," etc.
3. Net contents of the package in the same format as prescription drugs
4. A pregnancy-nursing warning on drugs intended for systemic absorption that advises any woman who is pregnant or nursing to get a physician's advice before taking the drug
5. Name and location of the manufacturer or packager

6. A listing of active and inactive ingredients
7. The amount and frequency of each dose and how it should be administered
8. Warnings indicating the limits of use, if any, the side effects, if any, and circumstances that may require a doctor's advice before taking the medicine
9. A description of the tamper evident feature incorporated in the package
10. The expiration date and the lot or batch code
11. So-called *label flags* which alert the customer to changes in the contents or to new warnings
12. The name of any habit-forming drug contained in the preparation

Of the twelve items listed above, all but #11 and the listing of inactive ingredients are required by law. Those two additional items are included in the industry's voluntary regulation program [15].

In addition to all this material, the OTC label must cover special situations with the following types of information:

- warnings against adverse interactions with other drugs
- telling the consumer to see a doctor if conditions do not improve
- information, such as sodium content, for consumers who may have special problems or conditions
- *keep-out-of-reach* warnings and advice on actions to be taken in case of accidental overdose

As always, the FDA is considering additional labeling requirements. With an eye to the aging population, the agency is now reviewing comments on a proposed rule that would require pharmaceutical manufacturers to inform physicians of their product's effects on elderly patients, specifically those over sixty-five, who constitute about 12% of the U.S. population but consume over 30% of prescription drug products and 40% of OTC drugs. Similar labeling is already required for children under age twelve. The thinking behind this proposed rule is, for example, that as kidney function declines with age, the body becomes less able to purge a drug from the system. For another example, older people are more likely to be on other medications that might adversely interact with the drug in question. The geriatric information required would be put in a separate section of the *precautions* section entitled *geriatric* use [16].

It may come as a surprise to learn that a pharmacist may legally repackage or relabel OTC drugs purchased in bulk. This is a risky business, since the pharmacist who relabels takes responsibility for compliance with CGMP, all the federal and state regulations, and the possible necessity to register as a manufacturer (if the repackaged items are sold to other retail establishments). Repackaging bulk products into unit doses by hospitals or pharmacists for in-house sale or dispensing does not carry these responsibilities [17].

THE NATIONAL DRUG CODE AND BAR CODING

The National Drug Code (NDC) has become a useful device for identifying each drug product with a unique, all-numeric number (as opposed to numbers and letters) that identifies the drug manufacturer/labeler, product and package size. Drug manufacturers offer, and drug wholesalers order, products using the NDC. Pharmacy computer systems, drug industry support systems, and third-party prescription claims processing, sales tracing, and reporting all use the NDC as a basis of identifying, describing and paying for pharmaceutical services. The law does not yet require the use of the NDC, but virtually every drug product label contains such a number.

USP is now considering recommending the use of a three-character identification code for solid dosage forms of drugs, vitamins and minerals. This code would be printed on individual tablets or capsules and would simply identify the drug, not the manufacturer or the strength. USP argues an important consumer benefit: when a prescription is refilled using a generic equivalent instead of a proprietary product, the buyer could verify the equivalence of the generic by comparing the codes, which must be the same for both [18].

Both the NDC and its bar code equivalent are too large to be printed on individual tablets or capsules. Nevertheless, USP proposed to establish a linkage between the two systems that can be tracked by a computer if necessary. USP's proposal is now in the second comment stage. Responses from manufacturers have expressed concerns of one kind or another, while responses from consumers and consumer groups were generally favorable. The proposal is being altered to reflect industry concerns and will likely be adopted soon on a voluntary basis [19].

The widespread use of the NDC provides a logical basis for the adoption of bar coding to identify drug products using the Universal Product Code format. A bar code is a series of black and white bars and spaces that represent a series of characters or symbols. Its purpose is to code information in a form that is readily read by a machine that sweeps a small spot of light across the symbol which must be large enough so that the light cannot wander outside its limits. Various formats have been adopted but the Universal Product Code (UPC) is appropriate to capture the information contained in the NDC, which covers most of the essential information needed to verify that a product has been correctly labeled.

The bar code is read by a scanner, which consists first of a light source, either incandescent or laser generated, and a detector which senses the light reflected from the coded section of the label and converts that information into a series of electrical signals which change as the intensity of the reflected light changes. This analog signal is decoded by measuring the time duration of each portion of the signal and feeding that data to a microprocessor which is programmed to compare the decoded pattern with the correct pattern and signal action to be taken (such as rejecting the incorrectly labeled article) if the inputs do not match.

The above is a simple description of what is in actuality a complex technology. For further information, the reader is referred to the literature or to suppliers.

Most drug packagers now bar code some of their products since bar coding offers many advantages:

- Input and collection of transaction data is automated, eliminating the error potential of manual keystroke entries.
- Efficient inventory management is enhanced.
- Manufacturers' processes that depend on positive identification of container contents become faster and more accurate, and labeling errors can be reduced.
- Both wholesalers and pharmacies gain efficiency in the entire range of individual operations that take place when a drug goes in and out of these institutions.

The only significant negative is the space that a functional bar code requires on an already crowded label. This problem becomes particularly acute in the case of unit dose labels, so much so that only recently has any supplier bar coded unit dose packages on each dose [20]. Although a stacked bar code would probably be best for very small packages like blisters, adoption of that system is still in the future since scanner and verifier changes are necessary. Thus, the first bar coded blister uses Code 128, the smallest possible symbology compatible with existing readers. It is so small that only the NDC number can be included—the expiration date and lot numbers are missing.

Bar coded unit dose packages have many advantages in hospitals, where the nurse could scan a bar code on the patient's wrist band and the bar code on the package to verify that the medicine was the correct one. Some hospitals have reported important savings when they applied bar codes to blisters. Bar coding by the manufacturer would certainly be preferable to the hospitals doing it themselves.

Experts in the field estimate that as of mid-1991, about 60% of primary container labels are bar coded but only about 5% of the distribution system is fully set up to take advantage of these bar codes [21]. This 5% is expected to become 60–80% in the next five years.

The reader interested in pursuing this aspect further is urged to consult a booklet available from the National Wholesale Druggist's Association: *NWDA Background and Position on Numerical and Automatic Identification of Drug Products*, NWDA, 105 Oronoco St., Alexandria, VA 22313.

LABELS AND THE LABELING PROCESS

Label Types

Drug package labels can be classified into three broad categories: glued paper, self adhesive (also known as pressure sensitive), and heat sensitive. Of these three, the first category, which is also the oldest, is rarely found in drug labeling operations today due largely to the mess that glue creates when used in conjunction with high speed automated equipment on which uptime is at a premium. The second and third categories share the drug applications market about equally, but pressure sensitive types are expected to capture an increasing share of the market in the future.

Self Adhesive (Pressure Sensitive) Labels

These consist of the printed label, either paper, PVC or polyester, a layer of adhesive which is permanently and aggressively tacky when dry, and a transparent silicone-coated backing sheet which allows the adhesive-coated label to be wound up on a roll. The adhesive layer, which used to be solvent-based, is now usually a water-based acrylic or rubber-based latex composition which can be tailored for degree of tack (which allows peelability if desired), water removability, low or high temperature adhesion, UV light resistance and general weatherability. Care must be exercised in adhesive selection to avoid components that could migrate through the wall of a plastic container and contaminate the drug package contents. At the same time, it is crucial that the adhesive must be powerful enough to strongly resist label loss or switching that could cause an unwary consumer to take the wrong drug.

Pressure sensitive label stock is almost always manufactured by companies specializing in this activity. After the three layers have been assembled, the paper and adhesive layers are die cut to allow for later separation of the individual labels in the labeling machine. They are then shipped in roll form to the drug manufacturer or labeler.

The continuous, automatic machine that applies these labels to the container consists (Figure 7.1) of an unwind station where the roll of label stock is fed around a stripper plate or peeler bar over which it reverses direction almost 180°. This sharp bending action causes the backing sheet to peel away from the die cut label array, freeing each separate label for pickup by the container. The backing sheet can then be separately wound up on another roll for eventual disposal. Each label is then either:

- picked up by a container by its leading edge and moved past a pressure plate or plates which press the label firmly in place

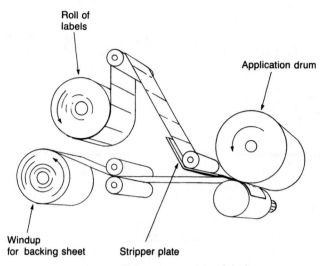

FIGURE 7.1. Pressure sensitive labeler.

- picked up by a vacuum head, positioned over the container, and pressed in place by an air jet which replaces the vacuum, or
- picked up by a vacuum drum and applied to the container in one continuous motion

It should be obvious that this is a greatly oversimplified description of a complex operation which must include machinery that assures that the containers are in the right place and correctly oriented.

Initially much higher cost than glue labeling, self adhesive label costs have been steadily reduced to the point that although they are still roughly twice as expensive as plain paper labels that must be glued on, the simplicity, speed, cleanliness and low maintenance features of this process have made it far more popular than glue labeling [22]. Speeds now exceed 600 labels per minute. Dual head machines have been introduced which apply both back and front labels simultaneously. Dual heads have been placed in series that allow automatic switching from an exhausted to a fresh label roll. Fan folded labels stored in cartridges can be substituted for rolls, allowing two or more label lengths to be connected end-to-end before machine startup, thus lengthening the run before shutdown [23].

As time passes, pressure sensitive systems will continue to grow in drug package labeling at the expense of heat seal systems, due largely to the relative simplicity, efficiency and operational ease of pressure sensitive labeling equipment [24].

Heat Seal Labels

As their name implies, heat seal labels require the application of heat to activate the adhesive, which can be LDPE, EVA, or PVC copolymers. These adhesives when cool are not tacky and therefore require no backing sheet to enable the coated labels to be wound on a roll. Thus the cost of these labels is generally lower than the cost of pressure sensitive labels, a cost saving that is offset by the higher cost of the equipment required to apply them [24]. For heat-sensitive products, such as some foods and drugs, the adhesive can be formulated in a so-called *delayed action* mode in which the application of heat converts the adhesive to a pressure sensitive form so that heating equipment never comes near the product being labeled. This mode has the additional advantage that the heating elements need not have complex shapes to conform to irregular container shapes and surfaces.

Heat seal labels have the additional advantage of providing a more secure labeling system, since heat activated adhesives usually provide a stronger bond to the container wall.

The automatic machinery that applies heat seal labels to containers consists of a station that holds the roll of labels from which they are cut off and fed to a heated vacuum drum. This drum contacts the container and rolls with it, pressing the label against the container wall. The pressure and dwell time required in this step are both greater than in pressure sensitive labeling. The alternative to this process is *flagged-on* labeling, which is used for containers that are not cylindrical. Here the heated label is pressed on the container along a label edge. As the container then travels down the belt, cold pads press the rest of the label in place. As with delayed action heat seal labels, this technique avoids heating the pressure pads which must be specially contoured to fit the irregular container contour [25].

Throughout this discussion, we have stated that the label feed to the process is in the form of rollstock. While this is not always true, the FDA urges, and may eventually require, that rollstock rather than cut labels be the feedstock, since the possibility of label mix-up is much higher with cut labels.

Common to all types of labels is the growing complication of package recycling. A PVC label on a PET container, for example, may well impede the recycling of the PET container unless the label can be easily removed. Recycling considerations are also affecting the choice of label material in another way: the public perception that paper is readily recycled and the ready availability of recycled paper are both boosting the popularity of recycled paper labels [26].

NONCONTACT CODING

Two methods are now in use for marking packages, including drug containers, in a way that does not depend on physical contact between the container and the marking machinery: ink-jet printing and laser coding. Both methods are being increasingly used because they are independent of surface texture and configuration. For example, an ink-jet printer can readily mark a ripe peach; a laser can mark a surface that will not accept inks. Both will place codes over rough and uneven surfaces.

Ink-Jet Printing

In its simplest form, an ink-jet printer ejects a continuous fine stream of ink through a nozzle and then through an ultrasonic device that breaks up the stream into a series of attached droplets. This stream is broken into individual droplets by mechanical and electrostatic forces as they pass through a positively charged tunnel. In the tunnel, the droplets are given varying degrees of electrostatic charge, the strength of which governs the extent of deflection they experience as they subsequently pass over a negatively charged deflector plate. This varying deflection sets the pattern they form when they strike the surface to be printed. A computer program controls the charge applied to each drop, so the printed pattern can be changed by a keystroke operation.

This technique has the advantage of great mechanical simplicity and is used in drug packaging for lot numbering, expiration date coding, and consecutive numbering. It is particularly well suited for such uses because the information printed can be programmed to be different for each container that the printer senses without incurring the cost and complexity that would be involved were each label to be uniquely printed by a converter and then later mated to the correct container. Obviously, this technique is applicable to applying bar codes on containers and cartons [27].

Laser Coding

A laser is a beam of tightly focused, collimated light waves created by a high voltage charge of electricity passed through a tube containing various gases. When this energetic beam strikes a paper, plastic or painted surface, the paper, plastic or paint is instantly vaporized. If the subsurface is a laser-resistant material such as metal, it remains, making the contrast between the etched and unetched surface clearly evident. A pattern can then be created by passing the beam through a brass stencil and then focusing it before it strikes the surface to be printed.

Since this technique is very fast, it is readily adapted to creating sharp, nonblurred images at container line speeds in excess of 600 per minute. The imprinted code is more permanent than ink and can consist of characters as small as one-sixteenth of an inch. Since a laser beam is light, mirrors can be used to alter its direction and it can be focused with lenses. The systems are highly reliable and require almost no operator attention. To date, they are little used for pharmaceutical package labeling, cost being the major deterrent [28].

INSERTS AND OUTSERTS

As noted earlier, the extensive information that must be supplied with some drugs requires the frequent use of inserts and outserts. As the names imply, inserts are printed matter that is inserted within a box that also contains the primary drug package. Outserts, a strange but highly descriptive word that must have been coined by a pharmaceutical drug packager, consist of the same printed matter that is attached to the primary container without a box. Attachment can be effected by adhesives of the types discussed above, by double sided tape, or by plastic banding or overwrap, usually with a shrink film.

Before the days of plastics, boxes, sometimes with dividers, that helped avoid breakage of glass containers were common. The advent of shatterproof plastic containers and the concept of outserts combined to dramatically shrink the frequency of box use and lower packaging costs significantly.

After the editorial matter has been approved by the FDA, the insert/outsert is printed and delivered, either precut and folded or on a roll, to the packaging line which feeds the insert to an on-line cutting and folding step. Since the law regards the information on inserts/outserts to be as essential as the information on labels, the possibility of error while mating the insert/outsert with the container must be reduced as far as possible and with the same dedication that is applied to elimination of labeling errors. For this reason, roll-fed, rather than precut inserts and outserts, are preferred.

An elegant way to handle these complexities is the so-called *Fix-a-Form* technique recently imported from the U.K. Here the outsert is printed in small, crisp type on thin paper, fan-folded and adhered to the center of a flat, pressure sensitive label by extending the outer panel and using this extension to hold the adhesive. The combined label is spooled and fed to the labeling machine and attached to the container just as if it were a simple pressure sensitive label. If both parts of the label are bar coded, scanners can ensure that the right outsert is mated with the right label. Spooling minimizes the chance of mislabeling in the pharmaceutical plant. The pharmacist generally peels off the outsert, exposing an area that can carry the information he needs to provide.

The higher cost of this combined label is offset by the much simpler and faster labeling operation in the drug plant (no banding, no shrink tunnel, etc.) and the esthetics are reportedly superior. One large drug company has adopted this system for its penicillin and cephalosporin products [29].

LABELING ERRORS

To quote a recognized expert: "Of all the things that can go wrong during the production of a drug product, the one that occurs most consistently is applying the wrong label" [30]. Not only is mislabeling the most frequent problem, it is also the most dangerous one because of the obvious potential for injury or death.

In spite of increasing attention from both manufacturers and the FDA, the problem will not go away, as shown by the data in Table 7.1 [31].

To put these numbers in perspective, all categories of mislabeling accounted for about 25% of the total number of recalls every year in the period 1983–1988.

Although the data peak in 1988, in part because the number of 1987 cases led to increased inspection emphasis, the decline over the next two years is not impressive: about 25% [32]. Furthermore, it is instructive to look beyond the numbers at some of the mislabeling situations that prompted Class I recalls (the most serious category):

- Bottles of camphorated spirits intended only for external use were labeled as castor oil.
- Bottles labeled quinidine sulfate and intended for use in control of irregular heartbeat actually contained dicyclomine hydrochloride, an antispasmodic used to relieve intestinal cramps but totally ineffective in controlling life-threatening irregular heartbeat problems.
- An OTC cold medicine bottle contained instead a potent tranquilizer fatal to children.
- A prescription diuretic was mislabeled as a calcium channel blocking agent used to relieve angina.
- Four thousand bottles of propranolol hydrochloride, a heart drug, contained an antibacterial used to treat intestinal parasites [33].

In 1988, the FDA looked closely at the files and reports of the

Table 7.1. Mislabeling recalls by type.

Type	'83	'84	'85	'86	'87	'88	'89	'90	Total
Label Mix-Ups	7	8	9	11	16	25	10	8	94
Product Mix-Ups	5	8	8	6	3	10	8	13	61
Print Errors	0	10	7	9	3	3	6	15	53
Container Errors*	3	8	8	4	3	10	9	6	51
Insert Mix-Ups	3	0	1	4	0	2	2	2	14
Other	1	3	0	3	6	9	7	4	33
Totals	19	37	33	37	31	59	42	48	306

*Correctly labeled immediate package is placed in wrong intermediate container or shelfpack.

recalls to get at the root causes of the problem and recommend corrective action via regulation. This study focussed on label mix-ups, as opposed to product mix-ups. Product mix-ups are also an important problem but are not a labeling issue and must be attacked by better stock control.

The study results are presented in great detail in the Lord article [33] and in summary form on page 26394 of the June 23, 1989, *Federal Register* [34].

The causes most frequently encountered were the use of cut labels as opposed to rollstock; the use of labels of similar size, shape, and color to label different products; deviations from existing CGMP requirements; the use of undedicated packaging lines and packaging one lot of product under several different private labels.

Three good label control practices were never used in these recall situations:

- the use of labels differentiated by size, shape and color
- the use of dedicated packaging lines
- the use of electronic label verification systems that validate the labeling of each product (100% inspection)

Proposed CGMP changes still under review but expected to become final in 1993 that were developed as a result of this study are [34]:

- Prohibition of gang printing of labeling to be used for different drug products or the same product at different strengths or net contents *unless* the labeling so printed is adequately differentiated by size, shape, or color.
- Allow use of cut labels *only* if labeling and packing lines are dedicated to each different product or product strength, or 100% inspection is conducted by appropriate electronic or electromechanical equipment. This rule suggests that the use of roll labels *per se* will cure the loose label mix-up problem, but that is not necessarily so. The label printer, who may be unfamiliar with CGMP, may splice together two rolls which look identical on casual inspection but which may differ in potency [35].
- Exempt packagers from the requirement for label reconciliation *if* a 100% drug product label inspection is

employed during or after completion of finishing operations. This provision is basically a sweetener to make the conversion to 100% inspection more palatable to those packagers who are not yet set up for it. In fact, the FDA argues that this provision will result in cost savings for manufacturers who are already set up for 100% inspection but who now must also carry out reconciliation.

Reconciliation is defined as "procedures . . . [that] reconcile the quantities of labeling issued, used, and returned, and [that evaluate and investigate discrepancies] when [they] are outside narrow preset limits based on historical operating data" [36]. If the packager does not use some form of 100% inspection, either manual or electronic, reconciliation is essential. It will not of itself tell what went wrong, but rather it triggers a 100% inspection of the product of the run that failed reconciliation. In that 100% inspection, the error—mislabeling or a missing label—can be found. However, since reconciliation is essentially a counting procedure, it will not pick up cases where the correct number of labels have been provided but there is an error on any of those labels.

- Require manufacturers to have a *written* procedure that covers the identification and handling of filled containers that are not immediately labeled. The identification required must enable the determination of name, strength, quantity, lot, or control number, and expiration date. In an ideal world, labeling would immediately follow filling, but such a requirement would be impractically difficult for many packagers, particularly those dealing with many different products and many short runs. This provision is the closest the FDA can come to that ideal state.

The FDA does not regard these changes as having a significant cost impact. For example, the cost of a machine vision system in 1988 was about $40,000 [37]. The agency argues that since the number of mislabeling recalls will diminish, recall costs, which are certainly well above $40,000, will be saved.

When the information on recalls and the important role labeling errors played in those recalls became known to the industry, drug companies and packagers responded by moving in the directions signalled by the FDA's analysis of the data. Their major technological (as opposed to procedural) emphasis was the increasing adoption of automatic, electronic, or electromechanical on-line inspection and verification systems. Usually this was accomplished by using bar coding. As noted earlier, industry sources estimate that over 60% of primary packages are bar coded.

Bar coding coupled with automatic 100% inspection systems can be used in a variety of ways to reduce labeling errors. For example, packagers like to avoid short runs, but when faced with small orders, short runs are inevitable unless a large run can be made and the product not immediately sold can be stockpiled. Stockpiled product cannot be immediately labeled because it may be a private label product which ultimately will receive one of many different labels. Yet the packaged product must be unambiguously, immediately and permanently identified. One good solution is to affix a bar code, often on the bottom of the container, which can later be read to identify the contents and also be useful to customers [38].

A more typical example may be the company that bar codes its labels in a way that identifies the product inside the labeled container, runs the labeled container past a scanner that verifies the presence of the label, then reads the bar code to verify that it is the correct label for that product. The machine does this by shining light on the entire bar coded section and noting in the reflected beam a pattern of diminutions in intensity. This pattern is sensed by a rectangular array of tiny sensors, each of which convert what they see into an electronic signal whose pattern is then the same pattern as the bar code. These signals are sent to a master unit and compared with the correct signal which has been loaded into the system before the labeling run begins. These systems react so rapidly, compared to the speed of the moving container, that there is time to reread the label several times if necessary to be sure that the original reading was correct.

A less sophisticated *blob scanner* can also verify that the label carries a lot number and an expiration date, although such scanners cannot actually read what is written on the label.

A *gate*, which allows correctly labeled containers to pass and shunts off incorrectly labeled ones, completes the heart of the installation [39].

Systems such as these can also be designed to read not only bar codes, but actual text as well [40]. Nevertheless, many packagers stop short of systems that can read bar codes and are content to let blob scanners verify simply that a label is present and correctly oriented on the container. While this is better than manual reconciliation systems, as time passes more and more packagers will use more comprehensive systems [41].

THE DRUG PRODUCT PROBLEM REPORTING PROGRAM

The vigilance of the FDA is supplemented by this program, a voluntary effort operated under the joint sponsorship of USP, the FDA, the ASHP, and state pharmacy associations. Under the program, practicing pharmacists throughout the country report problems found with drugs in connection with performance, appearance, stability, packaging or labeling. Information received through this program has led to revisions in standards as well as corrective actions by drug companies, including recalls. Many thousands of reports are filed every year under this program [42].

Scrutiny of these reports by concerned professionals has led to suggestions for improving labeling of prescription drug packages by manufacturers. The salient recommendations are as follows [43]:

- Drug identity and strength should be the most prominent item on the label. The manufacturer's name and logo should be placed at the bottom. The authors (Davis and Cohen) point out that while the prominence of the manufacturer's name and logo may have some merit or significance in the marketing of OTC drugs, a pharmacist or a nurse is interested only in what is in the container, not who makes the product.
- Avoid label clutter by eliminating unnecessary verbiage, such as *brand of, handy 100s, prescription package,* etc.
- Avoid naked decimals (e.g., .5) and unnecessary use of 0 after a decimal, as in 100.0. The former can easily be read as 5 and the latter as 1000, especially in dim light.
- Always print on opaque surfaces. Printing directly on glass can be difficult to read.
- Avoid look-alike labels for dissimilar products. The

authors cite eight dispensing errors that are directly attributable to look-alike labels [44].

LABEL LEGIBILITY AND UNDERSTANDABILITY

Even absolute 100% accuracy in label identity and placement will not cure all the problems that beset pharmaceutical labeling. At least two remain: labels are not always sufficiently legible, and the text of the label is often too complicated for many readers to understand.

Label Legibility

Several organizations have addressed themselves to this issue, action which is particularly timely because of pending legislation in California that would require 10-point type on labels to make them more legible for senior citizens and the visually impaired [45]. Trade groups managed to convert this initiative to less offensive legislation which requires manufacturers to report to the legislature on how they will solve the problem.

One study of legibility from the standpoint of the elderly showed that the study group favored larger print, avoidance of italics, black-on-white rather than black-on-yellow, and a matte rather than a glossy surface [46].

Since this is largely an OTC issue, the Non-Prescription Drug Manufacturer's Association (NDMA) has developed guidelines for legibility. They point out that complex language is frequently mandated by the FDA and thus the manufacturers cannot always make it simpler on their own, and that slack fill restrictions imposed by federal law preclude the use of a larger container that would allow making the label larger. They then give a number of practical suggestions to label designers [47]:

- Avoid long lines of type and break up long lines by using several columns.
- Use frequent paragraphing.
- Avoid justification of type at the right-hand margin. This practice leads to frequent hyphenation.
- Use boldface, color highlights, and boxing for emphasis and to break copy into manageable segments.

- Use bulleting (as in this text) to again break up copy into manageable segments.
- Avoid upper case lettering where possible.
- Use 4.5-point type when printing black on white or 6-point if white on black.
- Use sans serif type.
- Leave ample space between letters, lines, and paragraphs.

These and other guidelines contained in NDMA's work should help solve the legibility problem.

ASTM has a committee working on standards to enhance identification of drug names on labels. Part of their efforts have been devoted to the problem that many label critics have identified: all drug labels from a given manufacturer look the same. Their recommendations, in draft form in late 1991, deal with label shape and color, type layouts and text face that each manufacturer could use to separate groups of drugs that have different actions or potency. Each drug group, in other words, would have labels that would be distinctive in respect to those four features.

In addition, they comment on colors (avoid pastels) and color contrasts and on the way in which the drug name and strength can be printed to maximize emphasis on these crucial pieces of information [48].

ASTM also has four standards that pertain to various other facets of drug labeling: small volume parenterals (D4267-89), user applied labels in anesthesiology (D4774-88), prefilled syringes (D4775-88), and solutions for dilution (D5022-89). The standard on small volume parenterals, for example, deals with label contents, type size, type orientation and legibility, including a standard test for determination of legibility.

These standards may be ordered from ASTM, 1916 Race St., Philadelphia, PA 19103.

Label Content and Understandability

The increasing threat of lawsuits over products that do not carry proper warnings on their labels concerns many industries besides pharmaceuticals. One behavioral research firm has studied drug package inserts and finds [49]:

- Most warning documents require a postgraduate degree to be fully understood.

- Many warnings appear after the first page which 50% of readers never go past.
- Warnings urge patients to consult their physician when in doubt, but few do.
- Formatting doesn't separate the crucial from the trivial.
- Warnings are not strong enough, e.g., they use *should* instead of *must*.
- Warnings such as *periodically check for . . .* are ambiguous, e.g., How often is *periodically?*
- Text and diagrams contradict one another.

A more recent study, after pointing out that ". . . OTC labeling regulations require that labeling be stated in terms that are likely to be read and understood by the average consumer, including those of low comprehension . . ." and that the FDA believes that clear labeling precludes counseling on use of OTC products, describes a recent investigation that indicates problems in the comprehension area [50]. For example, a pediatrics panel concluded that a selected group of 500 mothers observed over a nine-month period had done "slightly more harm than good" in administering OTC medications to their children by relying on guesswork rather than on label instructions. As another example, a study of pharmacists revealed that only 3% felt that their customers were qualified to choose OTC products without professional advice.

To study label comprehensibility further, the authors of this study subjected twenty-one product labels to the Fry Readability Graph and the Fog Index. They found that only one label could be comprehended with only a seventh-grade reading level. Over half required a tenth-grade level or higher and six required a college education. Yet *half* the adults in the U.S. are reading below the tenth-grade level and 20% are functionally illiterate.

In addition to lack of communication stemming from inadequate comprehension, the group analyzed label instructions to see if they were clear and unambiguous. Some were not.

To evaluate label readability, an optometrist studied twenty-five OTC labels and found that in most cases, a visual acuity of 20/50 was adequate to read the label when it was held between 14 and 18 inches from the eyes. In some cases, 20/20 vision was needed. Holt et al. then note that a 1972 HEW study showed that only 72% of individuals between the ages of four and seventy-four had 20/20 vision in their better eye *with corrective lenses*. The results get worse when older segments of the population are singled out: only 33% of the population over age sixty-five has 20/20 acuity with corrective lenses.

It appears that OTC labels are not yet sufficiently readable and understandable to warrant the official conclusion that OTC packages are safely marketable without the aid of a healthcare professional.

In summary, it seems safe to assume that in view of the increasing attention being given to these drug labeling problems by consumer groups and by Congressional committees [51], drug labelers will continue to struggle with the problems of legibility, understandability, and completeness, even though some of the difficulties are not of their own making [51].

REFERENCES

1. A drug recall is rated Class I when there is a possibility that death could result if the drug was not recalled.
2. Densford, L. 1990. *Food and Drug Packaging* (December):4.
3. FDA. 1991. Title 21 of Code of Federal Regulations (CFR) (April 1):subparts A–G, sections 201.1–201.136, pp. 10–55.
4. Anon. 1991. *Food and Drug Packaging* (August):4.
5. FDA. 1991. Title 21 of Code of Federal Regulations (CFR), sections 201.56 and 201.57.
6. Ibid., sections 201.300–201.316.
7. 1990. *Pharmacy Law Digest*, p. DC-20.
8. Anon. 1988. *Food and Drug Packaging* (September):4.
9. 1979. "ASHP Guidelines for Repackaging Oral Solids and Liquids in Single Unit and Unit Dose Packages," *Am. J. Hosp. Pharm.*, 36:223.
10. Davis, N. M. and M. R. Cohen. 1983. *Medication Errors*. Philadelphia, PA: George F. Stickley & Co., p. 245.
11. 1990. *Pharmacy Law Digest*, p. DC-26.
12. Anon. 1985. *Am. J. Hosp. Pharm.*, 42:378.
13. 1990. *Pharmacy Law Digest*, p. DC-26.
14. Gennaro, A. R., ed. 1990. *Remington's Pharmaceutical Sciences, 18th Edition*. Easton, PA: Mack Publishing Company, p. 1569.

15. "Medicine Labels and You," NDMA Office of Public Affairs, 1150 Connecticut Ave., N.W., Washington, DC 20036.

16. 1990. *Federal Register* (November 1):46134.

17. 1990. *Pharmacy Law Digest*, p. DC-18.

18. Densford, L. 1991. *Food and Drug Packaging* (January):4; *Pharmacopoeial Forum*, 9-10/90.

19. Keith Johnson, USP, private communication, 1991.

20. Anon. 1991. *Packaging Digest* (May):28.

21. David Prins, National Wholesale Drug Manufacturers Association, private communication, 1992.

22. Kelsey, R. J. 1989. *Food and Drug Packaging* (September):16.

23. Kelsey, R. J. 1988. *Food and Drug Packaging* (January):10.

24. Sportello, L. 1989. *J. Packaging Technology* (October):228.

25. Andy Paul, New Jersey Machine Co., private communication, 1992.

26. Anon. 1991. *Packaging* (March):37.

27. Stys, L. J. 1991. *Interphex* (April 18):113; Anon. 1991. *Food and Drug Packaging* (October):11.

28. Anon. 1991. *Food and Drug Packaging* (October):11; Anon. 1990. *Food and Drug Packaging* (January):30.

29. Kelsey, R. J. 1990. *Food and Drug Packaging* (December):34.

30. Lord, A. G. 1988. *Pharm. Tech.* (May):50.

31. Anon. 1990. *Food and Drug Packaging* (December):32.

32. Anon. 1989. *Packaging* (November):9.

33. Lord, A. G., op. cit.; Densford, L. 1988. *Food and Drug Packaging* (March):3.

34. 1989. *Federal Register* (June 23):26394–26396.

35. Lee, J. Y. 1985. *Pharm. Manuf.* (September):35.

36. FDA. 1990. Title 21 of Code of Federal Regulations (CFR), section 211.125.

37. Lord, A. G., op. cit., p. 54.

38. Kelsey, R. J. 1988. *Food and Drug Packaging* (February):10.

39. Kelsey, R. J. 1988. *Food and Drug Packaging* (August):8.

40. Anon. 1990. *Packaging* (October):150.

41. Kelsey, R. J. 1989. *Food and Drug Packaging* (January):10.

42. Swarbick, J. and J. C. Boylan. 1988. *Encyclopedia of Pharmaceutical Technology*, Vol. 1. New York, NY: Marcel Dekker, p. 118.

43. Davis, N. M. and M. R. Cohen, op. cit., p. 88.

44. Ibid., p. 52.

45. Anon. 1991. *Chain Drug Review* (January 1):12.

46. Jinks, M. J., et al. 1990. *J. Geriatric Drug Therapy*, 5:55.

47. "Label Readability Guidelines," NDMA, 1150 Connecticut Ave., N.W., Washington, DC 20036.

48. ASTM. 1990. Third draft of "Proposed Standard Specifications to Enhance Identification of Drug Names and Labels," ASTM Committee D-10.34 (August 30).

49. Camden, C. and J. Wargo. 1986. *Food and Drug Packaging* (October):104.

50. Holt, G. A., et al. 1990. *American Pharmacy* (November):51.

51. Leary, W. E. 1992. *New York Times* (April 28).

CHAPTER EIGHT

Packages Used for Pharmaceuticals

In previous chapters each of the elements involved in packaging a pharmaceutical has been described: the characteristics of drugs and the various dosage forms, regulations, packaging materials, containers, closures and labels. In this chapter, all of these will be brought together by describing the primary packages used for pharmaceuticals. Here, package means the total system: the container, closure, liner, label, pumps, valves, etc.

The first part of this chapter describes the factors which must be considered in selecting or designing the package. Some of these determinants, such as product protection, are technical and are dealt with in quantitative terms while others, such as product image, are necessarily described qualitatively. For each determinant the discussion closes with an assessment of the relative importance it has in the package selection process.

In the second part, the interplay of these determinants is portrayed in the descriptions of current practice and trends in packaging the various dosage forms. The process of selection is further elucidated by explanations of the alternative choices available along with the advantages and disadvantages of each and with examples of problems—usually compatibility and stability issues—that have been encountered.

THE DETERMINANTS IN SELECTING OR DESIGNING A PACKAGE

The determinants to be described here are:

- product protection

- product/package compatibility
- FDA regulations
- product information
- product image
- consumer needs
- cost

Product Protection

Product protection is the level of protection demanded by the chemistry of the drug alone: its sensitivity to light, moisture and oxygen and its volatility or tendency to diffuse through the package. The drug must also be protected from chemical interaction with the package, but this requirement also involves the chemistry of the package and therefore is covered in the next section.

USP *Recommendations*

The USP is a primary source for recommendations of packaging specifications for each of the over 2000 drugs and pharmaceuticals listed. The package designations used by the USP are [1]:

1. *Well-closed container.* Protects the contents from extraneous solids and from loss of the drug under the ordinary or customary conditions of handling, shipment, storage and distribution. Maximum moisture permeability: 2000 mg per day per liter for 9 out of 10 samples measured; none may exceed 3000 [2].
2. *Tight container.* Protects the contents from contamination by extraneous liquids, solids, or vapors, from loss of the drug and from efflorescence, deliquescence or evaporation under the ordinary or customary conditions of handling, shipment, storage and distribution. Also it is capable of tight reclosure. Maximum moisture permeability: 100 mg per day per liter for nine out of ten samples measured; none may exceed 200 [2].
3. *Hermetic container.* Impervious to air or any other gas under the ordinary or customary conditions of handling, shipment, storage and distribution.
4. *Light resistant container* (also described as a container that offers protection from light). Protects the contents from the

effects of light by virtue of the specific properties of the material of which it is composed. Must meet light transmission specifications unless it is in an opaque enclosure. Specifications for glass: maximum percent transmission at any wavelength between 290 and 450 nm—10 to 50% depending on container size (from 1 ml to 50 ml) and type (flame sealed or closure sealed containers). For plastic (and type NP glass): maximum transmission 10% [3]. It is not stated why a higher percentage transmission is permitted for glass than plastic. Presumably since a higher percentage transmission is also permitted for flame sealed glass containers as compared to glass closure sealed containers, it is assumed that oxygen may also be a factor in any light-initiated reactions and hence the higher barrier packages need not be as light resistant.

5. *Single unit container.* Designed to hold a quantity of drug intended for administration as a single dose promptly after the container is opened. For oral solids, classes are established based on permeability. Class A: In nine out of ten samples tested, less than 0.5 mg of drug permeates the container per day and none exceeds 1 mg. Class B: nine out of ten less than 5 mg per day and none exceeds 10. Class C: nine out of ten less than 20 mg per day and none exceeds 40. Class D: none meet above standards. The same classes are used for unit dose [4].

7. *Single dose container.* A single unit container for articles intended for parenteral administration only.

8. *Unit dose container.* A single unit container for articles intended for administration by other than the parenteral route as a single dose, direct from the container.

9. *Multiple unit container.* Permits withdrawal of successive portions of the contents without changing the strength, quality or purity of the remaining portion.

10. *Multiple dose container.* A multiple unit container for articles intended for parenteral administration only.

The *USP* listings were analyzed to gain a sense of the complexity of the recommendations and the extent to which the recommendations restrict the choice of packages. The analysis is summarized in Table 8.1:

These observations can be made from the data in Table 8.1.

- For product protection, the situation is not highly complex. All but 33 of the 2144 drug entries fall into 35 packaging designations; 85% of all the listings fall into just 7 designations.
- For the majority of the drug entries, the package recommendations are not restrictive. The most prevalent categories were tight and well-closed containers with 70.3% of the entries. For the combination of tight and well-closed containers, 69.1% were tight containers. Light resistant containers were specified for 30.3% of the

Table 8.1. The distribution of drugs among the USP package designations.

Package Designation	Number of Listings	Percent
Tight	596	27.8
Tight + Light Resistant	444	20.7
Tight + Glass Only	3	0.1
Tight + Type I Glass Only	1	—
Tight + Glass + Light Resistant	1	—
Well-Closed	370	17.3
Well-Closed + Light Resistant	95	4.4
Well-Closed + Glass Only	1	—
Well-Closed + Single Dose Only	1	—
Container for Sterile Solids	124	5.8
Container for Sterile Solids + Light Resistant	8	0.4
Collapsible Tube	66	3.1
Collapsible Tube or Tight	39	1.8
Tube or Well-Closed + Light Resistant	13	0.6
Sterile Liquid for Injection, Glass Only:		
Single or Multiple Dose	33	1.5
Type I Only	108	5.0
Single Dose Only	44	2.1
Light Resistant	14	0.7
Type I Only + Light Resistant	33	1.5
Single Dose Only + Light Resistant	9	0.4
Single Dose Only + Type I Only	32	1.5
Single Dose + Type I + Light Resistant	34	1.6
Container for Sterile Liquid for Injection	24	1.1
Aerosol	18	0.8
Exceptions: Did not fit above designations	33	1.5
Totals	2144	99.7

entries. Thus one could meet the packaging recommendations for 70% of the entries by using a single package type that is both tight and light resistant, setting aside for the time being any concerns about product/package interaction and recognizing that many drugs packaged this way will be overpackaged.

- A minority of the drug listings have highly restrictive packaging requirements. Specific packaging materials are designated primarily for injections, which account for 15% of the entries. The nine categories of specifications for injectable fluids cover a range of restrictions from the least restrictive, "Containers for sterile fluids for injection," to the most restrictive, "Type I glass, single dose only, protect from light."

   The breakdown for injectable fluids packages was 30.2% specified Type I or II or Type I, II, or III glass, while 62.5% required Type I glass only and 7.3% listed just containers for sterile fluids for injection. "Single dose only" was specified in 36% of the entries. Outside the injectable fluids, specific packages were designated for only 10 other drugs (included in the group of 33 exceptions falling into none of the package designations in Table 8.1) which are especially volatile, corrosive, etc.

To determine just how broad the latitude of package choice is in practice for a given *USP* designation such as "tight container," it is necessary to evaluate the protection offered by a package. The next two sections cover such evaluation methods and the results for some typical packages.

Methods for Evaluating Package Protection

Some types of protection provided by a package can be determined adequately from measurements on the component materials as described in Chapter Four. Thus, resistance to light is straightforwardly determined by light transmission measurements on sections of the container and closure. Protection from gross contamination from the environment such as dirt is readily assured with almost any reasonable package. However, the barrier of the package to gases and to loss of product by diffusion is determined by the total package; not only by the properties of the separate components (container, closure, liner, membrane, cushioning, desiccant, etc.) but also by how they are assembled in the package (e.g., tightness of the closure). Knowledge of the separate component materials is helpful only as an initial screening to assist in establishing the most likely package alternatives. Final selection must be made on the barrier properties of the total package.

Moisture permeation is the most common problem. For oral solid drugs, loss of moisture can reduce cohesiveness between particles in the tablet, leading to crumbling and loss of potency; the tablet can also lose sheen. Gain of moisture may cause tablets to harden or soften, and disintegration times in the body can be altered.

In the moisture permeability test method described in the *USP*, a desiccant, typically calcium chloride, is carefully prepared and dried for reproducible results and placed inside the package [5]. The rate of weight gain for the drug and the package is measured at a controlled temperature and relative humidity. From this the moisture permeability is calculated and expressed as mg per day per liter. Since the package itself may also absorb significant moisture, it is necessary to also make determinations on empty packages.

Moisture pickup in a packaged drug can also be measured directly by determining the moisture content employing the Karl Fischer method which consists of dissolving the product in an appropriate anhydrous solvent and determining by titration the water content of the solution using a solution of iodine, sulfur dioxide, and pyridine in methanol. Another approach is to dry the moisture-laden, powdered product and measure the weight loss. Still another, more sophisticated technique involves the use of tritium-labeled water. By determining the level of radioactivity of the drug or desiccant, a direct measure of the rate of moisture absorption is obtained. This approach has the advantages of greater sensitivity and reduced time of measurement [6].

Measuring the permeability of a package with a standard desiccant gives a general performance rating which is based on how much moisture can penetrate the package. To know how much will actually penetrate that package containing a particular drug requires measurement of the specific drug/package system. In fact, the test must be made with the intended quantity of the drug in place since the permeation rate is dependent on the difference in the partial pressure of moisture on the outside and the inside of the package. The higher the rate of absorption of moisture by the product, the greater the differential. Thus, the amount of moisture taken up depends on both the inherent moisture sensitivity of the product and amount of product. Also, the rate of permeation changes over time as the moisture content of the drug product approaches saturation.

Instead of measuring directly the amount of moisture gained by drug products, the alteration of product effectiveness due to the chemical or physical interaction with moisture is also often used. Examples of this approach are studies on packaged efflorescent tablets. These products are formulated to generate carbon dioxide when mixed with water. Penetration of moisture into the package during storage of such tablets causes this same reaction and thus greatly diminishes or even eliminates effervescence on subsequent usage. This premature release of carbon dioxide in the package can cause an obvious pillowing of pouches which is a good qualitative indication of insufficient protection for many efflorescent products.

In a study of efflorescent potassium supplement tablets it was also found that tablets softened in the presence of moisture and that this effect could be used as a qualitative indicator of package failure, since softening correlated with the loss of effervescence. Also in this study, a dye test was used to identify minute imperfections in the foil structures used in these packages and a direct relationship was found between tablet instability and the number of such imperfections. The dye test consisted of removing the tablet through a circle cut in the pouch, swirling a few drops of dye solution inside the pouch and looking for the appearance of dye on the outer pouch surface [7].

Another moisture sensitive property of tablets which can sometimes be used to determine the effectiveness of package protection is the rate of dissolution of the tablet in water. In one such approach, dissolution rate was measured for tablets of prednisone, a steroid, stored in a variety of packages under a range of humidities and temperatures. For these particular tablets, moisture absorption leads to hardening and increased dissolution times. The dissolution rate was measured in the laboratory using exactly controlled conditions of stirring the tablets in water [8].

Results of Package Evaluations

The test methods described above provide two kinds of information useful in selecting packages with the appropriate level of product protection. The first is a moisture permeability rating allowing the package to be placed in a USP protection category (e.g., tight vs. well-closed). Second is a direct measure of product protection for a specific product/package system.

The moisture permeability rating of a package is calculated from the measurement of moisture gain using the USP procedures already outlined. As an illustration, Table 8.2 shows the USP classifications of several common multi- and single dose packages along with the measured permeabilities.

Knowing the USP classifications and permeability ratings for packages, it would seem to be a straightforward task to choose the optimum package for a drug using the USP recommendation for that drug. However, the selection process often doesn't follow this

Table 8.2. Packages classified by USP designations [8].

Package	USP Designation	Moisture Permeability
Prescription Vials		
PP Vial with HDPE Liner	Tight	30[a]
PS Vial with HDPE Liner	Well-closed	600[a]
Unit Dose Packages		
Strip Package:		
Foil/Paper Structure[c]	Class A	negligible
Bartuf Structure[d]	Class A	0.2[b]
Polyester-Paper/Foil[e]	Class B	3[b]
Blister Package:		
Copolyester-Paper/Foil[f]	Class B	0.6[b]
PVC Cup:		
PVC-Paper/Foil[g]	Class B	1.5[b]
Bag:		
LDPE	Class D	22[b]

[a]mg/day/liter.
[b]mg/day.
[c]Both webs: paper 0.5 mil PE on 0.35 mil aluminum foil/1 mil Surlyn.
[d]First web: 1 mil Bartuf 3 acrylonitrile copolymer/adhesive/1.5 mil Surlyn; second web: same as "c".
[e]Polyester sealed to paper-backed foil.
[f]6.5 mil copolyester/3 mil medium density PE sealed to adhesive/foil/paper.
[g]Saran-coated PVC cup sealed to paper/0.4 mil foil with silicone paper liner.

course. Drug manufacturers, repackagers and pharmacists generally want to minimize package inventories and avoid the opportunities for mixups. These considerations plus the generally conservative attitude of the industry often lead to the use of a single, all-purpose package type such as tight packages for all oral solids even when the *USP* recommendations permit packages with lower levels of protection. However, where concerns about product protection are raised (especially for unit dose packages and products that are highly moisture-sensitive) the drug packager generally relies on tests of the specific drug/package system. This is especially important in establishing expiration dating.

An outbreak of concerns about product protection occurred in the early 1970s as a result of many drug decomposition reports that raised doubts about some of the new plastic packages. These concerns led to many published studies including a broad study of the permeability effects of specific packages by the Drug Research and Testing Laboratory at USP. While these USP results published in 1981 are now ten years old they represent a valid characterization of these currently used packages, and little work has since been published that relates package performance for a specific drug to the USP ratings of the packages. In this USP study, the effect of storage on dissolution rate of model prednisone tablets in various packages under a variety of conditions was determined using the techniques described earlier. The packages used were those shown in Table 8.2. The results of storage of these packages of prednisone tablets correlated in general with permeability ratings as can be seen in Table 8.3 [8]. Note that while fresh tablets dissolved to the extent of about 70%, after storage at 40°C and 75% RH for 8 weeks, the extent of dissolution varied from about 70% to as low as 43% depending on package permeability.

Package protection data for specific drug products are important not only for the selection of the optimum package but also in establishing the expiration date for the packaged drug. Where the effects of moisture are the determining factor in establishing the expiration date, it is necessary to establish how much gain or loss of moisture a product can tolerate before the minimum acceptable level of potency is reached or before the product has been so altered as to make administration not viable. An example of the latter would be tablets that stick together or even dissolve in the absorbed moisture. Once this point has been established, the product can then be tested in a package to determine the time re-

Table 8.3. Extent of dissolution of model prednisone tablets after storage in various packages at 40°C and 75% RH for 8 weeks.

Package	Percent Dissolved	Permeability
Initial	70	
Multidose Packages		
Tight Container	70	30[a]
Well-Closed	60	600[a]
Unit Dose Packages		
Class A (Foil/Foil)	74	negligible
Class A (Bartuf/Foil)	61	0.2[b]
Class B (Blister)	59	0.6[b]
Class B (Polyester/Foil)	53	3[b]
Class D (PE Pouch)	43	22[b]

[a]mg/day/liter.
[b]mg/day.

quired to reach it. It is apparent from studies like those on prednisone tablets that the package has a strong influence on shelf life. The USP declares ". . . the expiration date stated on the manufacturer's or distributor's package has been determined for the drug in that particular package and may not be applicable to the product where it has been repackaged in a different container" [9]. In fact, if a drug is repackaged the expiration date of the new package cannot exceed 25% of the remaining time (between repackaging and original expiration date) or six months beyond repackaging, whichever is shorter, unless stability data in the new package establishes that the original date is still valid [9].

Direct measurements of the shelf life of a particular drug/package system can be tedious and time consuming. On the other hand, shelf life prediction methods have been well established where moisture permeability is the limiting factor. The development of this science, which began with packaged food products, has continued over the past forty years. These efforts have led to mathematical and computer methods based on an equation that describes mass transfer across a membrane. With the critical moisture content of the drug (the point of minimum acceptable potency, etc.), the permeability of the package, and the conditions of storage (temperature, relative humidity) all defined, these methods can be used to predict the shelf life. The effectiveness of the prediction can be validated by a small number of selected actual measurements [10,11].

The Relative Importance of Product
Protection in Package Selection

In theory, product protection is the most significant determinant. The drug manufacturer's primary concern is that the drug product gives the consumer all of its benefits when it is used. Adding to this motivation are federal regulations and concerns about lawsuits stemming from product failures. In practice however, the vast majority of drugs do not have demanding protection requirements (such as an absolute barrier) as seen in Table 8.1. Also, there is usually a variety of alternative package possibilities for the level of protection required. Therefore, in practice, meeting product protection needs is generally not highly restrictive in determining package choice. This is reflected in the growing use of plastic packaging for all dosage forms but especially for oral solids, where 70–80% are in plastic bottles [12]. The exceptions to this generality are noteworthy, however, in that much attention has been given to them in packaging studies reported in the literature.

Compatibility

For product protection, USP recommendations are specific about package type since they depend only on the properties of the drug. By contrast, specific compatibility recommendations cannot usually be made since interaction of a drug with a package depends on the chemistry of both the drug and the package. But there are exceptions; for some injectable fluids, USP recommends "glass only" or "Type I glass only," etc. Among the 33 drugs that did not fall into one of the 35 general categories in Table 8.1, there are a few cases where specific restrictions related to compatibility are given: glass or PE, nonmetallic, plastic container and collapsible lined or coated tube.

Thus the packager has the responsibility to be certain that "the container does not interact physically or chemically with the article placed in it so as to alter the strength, quality, or purity of the article beyond the official requirements" [13]. While there are a few compatibility problems with glass (a prominent case being with nitroglycerine preparations) and with metal containers for corrosive drugs, the concern has been primarily with plastic packages. Beginning in the early 1970s many compatibility studies of drug/packaging systems were conducted. For sterile dosage forms, an excellent summary was published in 1984 by Wang and Chien. They summarize in one table the results of sorption studies on 115 different drugs [14]. A significant change (discoloration or 10% or greater absorption of the drug) occurred in 36% of the systems studied. While compatibility problems are considerably less common for other dosage forms, they have been encountered, and quantitative analysis of the problem is not always easy.

The term compatibility encompasses three different consequences of chemical interaction between the package and any of the components of a drug product formulation. The first results in actual reduction in drug availability or potency through sorption—the removal of the drug by the package. The second results in contamination as the formulation extracts substances from the package. The third causes breakdown of the package by deterioration of its strength, stiffness or barrier properties as the formulation chemically attacks the package.

Sorption

When formulation components are removed by a package two different processes are involved: adsorption onto the surface and absorption into the package wall by diffusion. A component may also desorb from the outer surface of the package and pass into the atmosphere if it is volatile enough. Strong adsorption or absorption requires a strong chemical interaction between the component and the packaging material. In addition, for a high level of absorption the packaging material must be permeable to the component. Glass has a chemically active surface but is an absolute barrier so that while adsorption can be strong, no absorption occurs. For plastics, on the other hand, both adsorption and absorption are possible. In the literature, when adsorption and absorption occur together, there is rarely a distinction made between the two and therefore the term sorption will be used to indicate both are taking place.

The usual method for measuring sorption is to soak a known quantity of the packaging material, usually a thin film or section of the container wall, in a solution of the drug product or in the formulation if it is a liquid. Either the amount of a component lost from the solution or the weight gain by the packaging material is measured. Of course, sorption studies of actual product/package systems have also been made. When a multicomponent formula is involved, separation of the interaction of the different components is much more complicated. In one example of a sophisticated technique used for this purpose, phenylephrine, a decongestant, was labeled with radioactive carbon and placed in PE nasal spray bottles. Concentration changes of the active drug alone were followed using internal liquid scintillation spectrometry which distinguished the phenylephrine interaction from those of the other components in the formulation [15].

There have been many studies of sorption kinetics leading to a number of different mechanisms and equations aimed at predicting rate of sorption and its dependence on key variables such as drug composition, plastic type, and temperature. However, as Wang and Chien conclude: "Given the conflicting results in the literature, it is difficult to predict sorption activity. It seems more appropriate, at this stage of knowledge, to study such activity, rather than try to predict it" [16].

Leaching

Leaching is primarily a problem with IV fluids and large volume parenterals. Widely studied examples are the leaching of plasticizers from PVC IV bags, extraction of additives from rubber closures and corrosion of glass surfaces. Most leaching problems occur with plastics because of the presence of additives such as fillers, activators and plasticizers. Leaching can cause discoloration, precipitation, change in pH, and contamination that can lead to increased toxicity or instability of the drug.

The *USP* describes several tests for leaching [17]. For glass, a powdered sample in purified water is autoclaved at 121°C and the water is then tested for the amount of alkali present. This test is used to confirm that a container intended for injectable fluids is made of the appropriate type of glass. For plastics, purified water at 70°C is used as the extracting medium for containers. The water is then examined for volatile, nonvolatile and heavy metal residues as well as acidity and alkalinity. In addition biological tests are performed in two stages: *in vitro* tests on cultures of mammalian fibroblast cells and *in vivo* tests on small animals. Materials that fail to meet the requirements of the *in vitro* tests must undergo *in vivo* testing. For the *in vitro* tests, plastic samples are extracted with saline solution at either 50°, 70°, or 121°C depending on the heat resistance of the plastic. The extraction medium is expanded to include polyethylene glycol, vegetable oil, drug product vehicle and water for the *in vivo* tests. Evidence of biological activity, as judged by visual observation, after contact of the extract with the cell culture or of adverse reaction after injection of the extract into animals, means failure. For plastic containers for ophthalmic fluids, the incidence of eye irritation in rabbits caused by extracts denotes failure [18].

In extraction tests, it is desirable to identify all the materials leached out. The detection of acidity, alkalinity and metal salts is straightforward but identification of organic molecules is much more difficult. Sophisticated techniques reported in the literature include UV spectrometry, mass spectrography, nuclear magnetic resonance, atomic absorption spectrometry, gas chromatography and thin layer chromatography. In one interesting example, a high performance liquid chromatograph was used to detect in levothyroxine sodium tablets (used to treat hypothyroidism) the presence of materials from the package. In this case, diethyl phthalate was found and its source was the PVC container used for the desiccant [19].

A number of different mechanisms and equations have been derived from leaching data, yet there appears to be little dependence on these equations for predicting results for systems not yet studied. Evaluations of specific systems of interest is the course most often followed.

Modification of the Container

The physical or chemical alteration of packaging materials by drug products is called modification. Permeation, sorption and leaching all can alter properties of plastics and may also lead to degradation. Some solvent systems have been found to be responsible for considerable changes in the mechanical properties of plastics. Oils, for example, soften PE and fluorinated hydrocarbons attack PE and PVC. Changes in PE caused by some surface active agents have been noted. In some cases, the drug formulation may extract the plasticizer, antioxidant or stabilizer and change the flexibility of the package. PVC is an excellent barrier for petroleum-based solvents but the plasticizer in PVC is extracted by solvents, leaving the plastic hard and stiff.

Stress cracking of the container occurs when fluid causes the container to slowly develop cracks, usually in areas of unrelieved stress induced during fabrication. This problem is particularly acute for polyethylenes and increases in severity with increasing density. Polystyrene is attacked by many chemicals which cause it to craze and crack and therefore is generally used only for dry products. Polypropylene does not stress crack under any circumstances and generally shows excellent resistance to chemicals. Good resistance to chemicals is characteristic also of PET and nylons.

Container modification is evaluated by measuring changes in physical properties and observing physical changes after exposure to the intended contents. For stress cracking, a notched plastic bar is suspended under load in a test liquid. The time required for the notch to propagate and the bar to break is measured.

The Relative Importance of Compatibility in Package Selection

Sorption can change product potency; leaching can cause pharmaceutical products to discolor, precipitate, change pH, and become contaminated; and container modification can lead to container breakdown and product leakage. Although any of these compatibility problems can be serious, alternative, problem-free systems can usually be found. General guidelines (such as those outlined above for various plastics) have been developed and reasonably adequate theoretical analyses are available to help avoid problems. However, this is not a black-and-white situation. Some loss in drug potency is acceptable. Minor incompatibility is sometimes tolerated if its harmlessness can be assured and there are sufficient offsetting advantages of the package system. One example is the PVC bag for IV fluids where the disadvantageous leaching of nontoxic plasticizer is offset by the advantages of shatterproofness and collapsibility of the bag versus the glass bottle alternative.

In summary, compatibility problems, though extensively studied in the exceptional cases, are not often encountered for the vast majority of packaged drugs. Such problems are especially rare for solids, the principal dosage form. Additives in plastics are rarely toxic. Nevertheless, compatibility testing must be part of the screening process for package alternatives.

Regulations

Governmental regulations that directly affect drug container options are discussed in detail in Chapter Three. Those that affect labeling are covered in Chapter Seven. Two other groups cover measures required for tamper evidence and to prevent child poisoning impact closure design. These are discussed in Chapter Six. In this section only general comments will be made to put government regulations as determinants in perspective with the other determinants.

The FDA must be convinced that the package for a specific drug will preserve the drug's efficacy as well as its purity, identity, strength and quality for its designated shelf life. It is the responsibility of the packager to prove the safety of a package and get approval before using it for any drug product. Data must be included on the container and package components in contact with the pharmaceutical product in the NDA. Once approved, there can be no significant alteration of the package without prior approval and even minor changes must be reported after the fact. A significant alteration could be a small increase in the area of a package in contact with the drug. Minor changes are things such as a change in the supplier of packaging materials where there is supporting data to establish the equivalence of the substitution.

While these regulations appear restrictive, it must be kept in mind that the FDA does not specify the packages or materials to be used. The regulations create a discipline by requiring the testing and generation of supporting data which, for the most part, a prudent manufacturer would normally undertake anyway to assure suitability of a proposed package. Later we will give examples of cases where this was not done adequately and the packages provided insufficient protection or presented compatibility problems. All these examples occurred in situations with minimum regulatory scrutiny, such as pharmacy repackaging as single units.

The regulatory process has an important indirect effect on restricting package choice for a new drug because it adds significant time and some uncertainty to the commercialization of the drug. The tendency is to resist introducing new, innovative packaging and to stick to conventional approaches. Similarly, changes to new packages for established products are inhibited by the time required for approval (usually about two years), the burden of additional testing and the paperwork required by the reporting regulations. Manufacturers are even reluctant to consider a change within a package that would open up for new scrutiny a package/drug system which was approved at a time when tests and regulations may not have been as stringent. Test requirements are continually changed and sometimes when a new package has been in the approval process for several years, the FDA suggests that the proposed package be retested according to the latest procedures. Given this regulatory environment, plus the innate conservatism of the industry, it is not surprising that even the largest companies with the technical resources to cope with the situation move cautiously.

Product Information

Another determinant in selecting or designing a package is the requirement to convey product information which the drug consumer needs to ensure the product is used safely and that its benefits are fully realized. The information that must be included is described in Chapters Three and Seven. The need to convey this extensive information by displaying it on the package and/or in an insert can affect its design. For example, for small packages such as tubes for ophthalmic ointments, a secondary enclosure, usually a carton, becomes mandatory to provide panel space and/or to contain an insert. In some cases, a larger sized primary package than that required for the product is used to provide a larger label and all the required product information. Clearly, this is not a critical determinant since such accommodations are relatively minor, especially when, for example, cartons are used anyway for the purpose of product image.

Product Image

The drug package contributes strongly by its design and its graphics to the impression the manufacturer wants to create for his product. Since the buyers are quite different for ethical versus OTC products, the approach in packaging is different.

Ethical products are handled largely by professional people—doctors, nurses, pharmacists, etc. Therefore the package image ideally reinforces confidence in the product by conveying professionalism in both appearance and function. As a result, ethical drug packages tend to keep color simple but positive.

By contrast, while occasionally a recommendation by a physician or pharmacist is made, the consumer generally makes the buying decision for OTC products. Therefore product image is critical, and drug manufacturers conduct market research to determine what the consumers' current impressions are. Conclusions from such data strongly influence graphics and package design. Key points are dramatized visually, and information is carefully selected to avoid overwhelming the package. Graphics are more decorative than for ethical packages with wide use of multiple color printing and pictorial representation. Cartons with flat panels ideal for printing are widely used. Product differentiation is sometimes sought through the use of novel package shapes and special convenience features. However, the manufacturer of drugs exercises far more restraint than do the food companies, lest the package become gimmicky and undermine consumer confidence and the image of ethical heritage.

Several examples will illustrate how product image is enhanced by a package. The first three are new OTC introductions of drugs that were previously sold only as ethical products. In each case, the package graphics underwent striking changes consistent with the change from a professional to a consumer market [20]. The package for Drixoral is shown in Figure 8.1. The best selling prescription cold tablet in the U.S., it entered the OTC market in direct competition with powerful incumbents: Contac, Teldrin, Dristan, Sudafed, NyQuil, and Allerest. Typically, the ethical package put primary emphasis on the manufacturer's name and subordinated the product name. On the new OTC package the product name dominated. Visual drama was achieved with a bull's-eye: a green tablet surrounded by a halo of white and then by a rainbow time clock, emphasizing 12-hour relief. Key points were prominent and concise: package content ("20 sustained action tablets"); product use ("antihistamine/nasal decongestant"); and benefits ("12-hour relief").

Also in Figure 8.1 is a sketch of the Phazyme 95 package. The unique feature of this tablet for relief of severe gas pain is that it is layered, allowing the separate release of simethicone in the stomach and in the small intestine. In the graphic design the product name was subordinated to the benefits ("For gas pain"). A

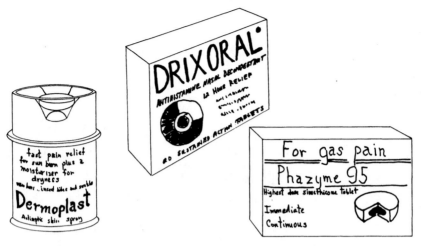

FIGURE 8.1. Enhancing product image in OTC packages.

picture of the layered tablet visually dramatized its dual-phase properties. Differentiation was emphasized by a strong message ("immediate . . . continuous . . . highest dose simethicone tablet") and supported by the red color of the tablet. Color was also used to set off the main messages boldly from secondary copy in smaller print.

In these two examples, cartons were used to carry the messages and graphics. In the next example, the container itself, an aerosol can was used. Dermoplast, an anesthetic skin spray created exclusively for in-hospital use, attained the top market position primarily as a sunburn remedy. In the OTC entry, the light beige color was chosen for differentiation from its competitors: Solarcaine, Rhulicaine, and Bactine. Its broad benefits were emphasized ("fast pain relief for sunburn plus moisturizer for dryness . . . for minor burns, insect bites, and scratches") along with the product name.

Unlike the examples above, Figure 8.2 shows two that are not new OTC introductions but are cases of product revitalization through changes in packaging. In the first case, the primary package for Maalox was redesigned to promote product differentiation while maintaining the pharmaceutical look. A standard round shape was chosen for the plastic bottle but a flip-top lid was added for greater convenience. The translucent HDPE container allows the consumer to see the unique two-piece tablets which are also simulated in the two-colored, two-piece closure [21].

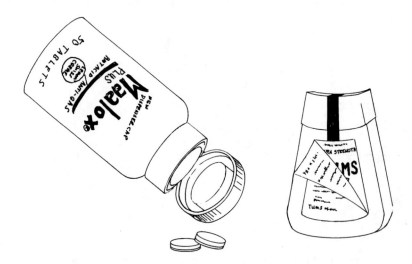

FIGURE 8.2. Enhancing product image in OTC packages.

For a new Tums container a distinctive, triangular-shaped, plastic bottle was chosen. An additional interesting approach was the use of a label that was also an instant redemption coupon to stimulate product awareness and repeat sales. For this purpose, two labels were used, one on top of the other, with the coupon portion to be removed, leaving the primary label intact [22].

While in most of the examples, product image was enhanced by a carton, there are many examples where product image is a strong determinant in selecting and designing the primary package. Convenience features, while also meeting consumer needs, are often chosen for differentiation. It seems likely that product image will continue to increase in importance, becoming a driver for manufacturers to more broadly adopt new packaging technologies that are commonplace in food packaging. Such technologies include PET bottles, multilayered plastic barrier containers and brick pack cartons. Package recyclability may also become a feature used to enhance differentiation.

Consumer Needs

Consumer needs include those aspects of the package that make it more consumer friendly. One of these is the presentation of product information in an easily readable and understandable form. The design of the label must accommodate this need and balance it with the needs for product image such as simplification and subordination of detailed product information. This subject is covered in Chapter Seven. As already mentioned secondary carton design and size are often dictated by such needs. Another approach is to use an insert or outsert.

Consumers, especially the elderly, also want packages that are easily opened and, for multiple unit packages, conveniently reclosed. Thus snap lids are preferred over screw caps. In the Maalox example, a hinged snap closure is used. Other closures are described in Chapter Six, as is the conflict between this desire for easy opening and the need for child-resistant and tamper evident features. An easy-open, easy-close feature can be seen in some cartons such as the one used for blister packs of Chloraseptic lozenges. Here it is a flip-top like the rigid cigarette box which clicks, insuring the user of a tight reclosure and enhancing portability [23].

Assuming the package is easily opened, the next consumer need is for the drug product to be conveniently dispensed. For solid, oral dosage forms, this need can be met by the use of large-mouth bottles. In the Maalox example, the package designers sought ". . . the largest orifice we could get" [20]. For multiple dose packages of liquids, there are many familiar examples of features that enhance convenient administration. These range from separate measuring cups for cold medicines to squeeze bottles for nasal sprays and ophthalmic drops, bottles with mechanical pumps including devices for control of dose size and aerosols with a dose control feature for inhalants. Squeeze bottles with hinged spouts are also used for dusting of topical powders. Unit dose would seem to be the ultimate in easy as well as confident administration of drugs. For tablets in blister packs each individual blister provides protection but the tablet can be readily removed. Easy portability is also achieved via perforations around each blister which facilitates tearing off the number of tablets desired. When Imodium antidiarrheal drug was switched from ethical to OTC in solid form as caplets, they were blister packaged. This approach greatly appealed to the travellers to whom the drug was promoted [24]. An excellent example of the convenience of unit dose packaging is seen in Snaplets medicated granules for children. These taste-free granules which are used to treat fevers, allergies, coughs, and colds are provided in easy snap-open

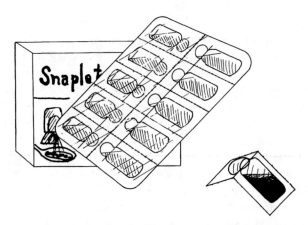

FIGURE 8.3. Example of convenience in administration.

blisters from which the contents can be sprinkled over soft food held in a teaspoon [25]. A sketch of the package is shown in Figure 8.3. The recent introduction of Robitussin cough syrup in easy-open blisters represents the first use of this package for liquids (see Figure 8.4).

It is evident from the many examples described above that consumer needs are becoming an increasingly important determinant in drug package selection and design. Meeting these needs often leads to proliferation of package types and to the broader use of

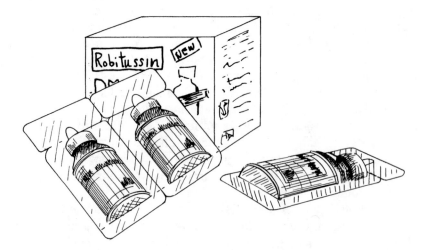

FIGURE 8.4. Single dose package for cough syrup.

plastic packaging versus glass or metal. Plastic overcomes the most basic disadvantages of glass such as heaviness and fragility. Furthermore, many of the convenience features are only attainable with plastic. Also for many applications, flexible packages offer the ultimate in consumer friendliness. As with product image, increasing attention to consumer needs will lead drug manufacturers to adopt the newer technologies in plastic packaging.

Cost

The package can play a significant role in affecting the profitability of drug products. Sales dollars, as discussed above, can be positively or negatively influenced by the package, especially for OTC products. Packaging cost is a significant part of total cost: about 10% of total product cost for ethical and as high as 50% for OTC products [26].

At this point it would be ideal to be able to present a detailed comparison of the costs of various drug packages. Unfortunately, cost numbers are rarely published. An example which is available gives the following comparison for packages of 30 tablets: glass bottle—$1.21; plastic bottle—$0.82 (materials $0.125, labor $0.70); blister pack—$0.31 (materials $0.07, labor $0.25) [27,28]. The savings for flexible packaging over a bottle are highest for the lower count packages with the break-even coming at roughly 100 tablets. In a report referring apparently to the same example, a drug firm is saving $500,000 per year by switching two of its OTC products from plastic bottles to blisters. Both involved 30-count packages [29]. In this example, the blister film was plain PVC, the lowest cost film for this application. As the level of moisture protection increases, higher cost structures are required. For example, PVDC-coated blister films cost twice as much as plain PVC. Aluminum foil laminates are three times the cost of PVC. Where both transparency and high barrier are required and ACLAR chlortrifluoroethylene films must be used, the cost is about ten times that of PVC film [30]. Even if material costs were doubled in the example above (recognizing that the materials costs are only partly for the blister component with the rest being the lidding structure), the total cost would still be only $0.38 per package and still greatly favor blister designs. The fact that labor savings account for most of the advantage in the cost of blisters over plastic or glass bottles is typical of flexible packaging with its higher degree of automation. Another labor saving example is the process used for packaging Romicol cough medicine cubes in thermoformed trays sealed with an aluminum/paper lid. Here, a separate cube-forming step was eliminated by pouring the liquid formulation directly into the tray where each tray section served as a mold for the solidifying product [31].

Despite such opportunities for profit improvement, package cost is not among the strongest determinants for package selection. The principal focus on other determinants like product protection and the time and effort required to qualify new packages are major deterrents to frequent package replacement.

Summary

Product protection and product/package compatibility depend on the chemical and physical properties of the product and the various components of the package. Most situations allow wide latitude in package choice and design; only a few restrict these choices to a narrow range. Governmental regulations dictate the discipline that the manufacturer must use in selecting a package and require substantial documentation of the appropriateness of the package. Also dictated largely by regulations is the product information which must be included on or within the package. This determinant, however, rarely affects package decisions beyond those governing size, labels and inserts. The last three determinants, product image, consumer needs, and cost, are under the manufacturer's control and can be brought to bear on the package decision once the choices are developed from the interplay of the first four. The results of applying this decision making process will be seen in the following descriptions of the packages used for the various dosage forms.

PACKAGES FOR SOLIDS

This discussion will begin by defining certain key terms for both solids and liquids:

Bulk packages refer to those used by the drug manufacturer to ship products to pharmacies or other repackaging operations.

Consumer packages are used for either OTC products or ethical products where the package is simply relabeled or placed in a secondary container (e.g., a carton) by the pharmacist and sold directly to the consumer.

Pharmacy packages are those used in the pharmacy to repackage dosage forms or to package a formulation prepared in the pharmacy.

Bulk Packaging

Large quantities of solids are usually packaged in drums made of metal, fiber or plywood or in multiwall paper bags or heavy-duty plastic bags. Drum lids are metal or plastic. Smaller quantities are packaged in bottles, cardboard cartons, boxes, or metal containers. An inner layer of plastic is often used in the latter three cases to overcome compatibility problems or provide protection from moisture. Such layers can be bags made of PE, PP or PVC, extrusion coatings or rigid, blow molded PE inserts. One of the classic protection problems is penicillin, which becomes totally inert unless packaged in containers with a high moisture barrier.

Bag-in-box, long used in food packaging for liquids, is being promoted for use with pharmaceutical solids, especially in combination with vacuum packaging techniques. This approach saves space and with the removal of head space gases can provide improved protection [32].

The maximum quantity packaged in bulk must be limited for some solids. For granules and uncoated tablets, the weight of the contents, if too large, will crush those in the bottom of the container. Larger diameter tablets break more readily than smaller ones. For example, 10.5 mm diameter aspirin tablets can be safely packaged in units of 50,000 whereas 12.5 mm codeine tablets must be limited in count to 5000 to 10,000. Coated tablets require no such limitations.

Consumer and Pharmacy Packages

Powders and Granules

Powders and granules include oral, topical (dusting powders) and sterile powders for injections.

For oral powders, multiple unit packages are usually bottles with wide mouths that facilitate dispensing. Plastic is often used but glass is recommended for especially moisture sensitive products and where volatile components can be lost. Sometimes spiral wound cylinders are used. Effervescent granules require a package with moisture barrier.

The single unit pharmacy package for powders has traditionally been prepared extemporaneously by folding bond paper or parchment. This is still the recommended procedure for packaging a preparation such as captopril, used for the treatment of pediatric hypertension, where the commercially available tablets are crushed and diluted by the pharmacist [33]. However, pouches or sachets, with their greater convenience and increased protection, are being used more and more by pharmacists. For consumer packages, single unit packages such as pouches, strip packages, and blisters are increasing in usage. The flexible webs are designed to provide the degree of protection required. An example of a single dose package is a cold remedy powder supplied in a packet. The required dosage is easily prepared by dissolving all of the contents of the packet in hot water. Metamucil therapeutic natural fiber is also packaged in this way. Another example is the Snaplets product described earlier where granules are contained in blisters that are easily broken open for dispensing the contents over soft food.

For the pharmacist, powders that are unstable in water are sometimes supplied, for greater convenience and accuracy, in screw cap bottles with just enough powder to provide a quantity of suspension or solution, when mixed in water, that maintains potency over the period of usage by the patient.

The traditional multiple unit package for topical powders is a metal can with a cap that can be rotated to expose holes. These have been largely replaced by plastic squeeze bottles, which are often equipped with a hinged spout to better direct the spray of powder. A typical application is the packaging of undecylenic acid or one of its salts for the treatment of athlete's foot. Aerosols are also used to package topical powders such as antibiotic preparations for burn treatment. Single unit packages for topical powders are rarely used.

Sterile powders for use in injections are always packaged in glass bottles or ampules. Containers must be sterilized and the closure system must be an absolute barrier to contamination. Biologicals, which are unstable in solution, are a good example of this category. They are provided as lyophilized (freeze-dried)

powders in hermetically sealed ampules or rubber-capped vials
[see Figures 8.5(a) and 8.5(b)] and are reconstituted by the introduction of an appropriate solvent. In one approach, lyophilization is accomplished by placing in a vacuum chamber the container with the stopper inserted only partway and then pushing

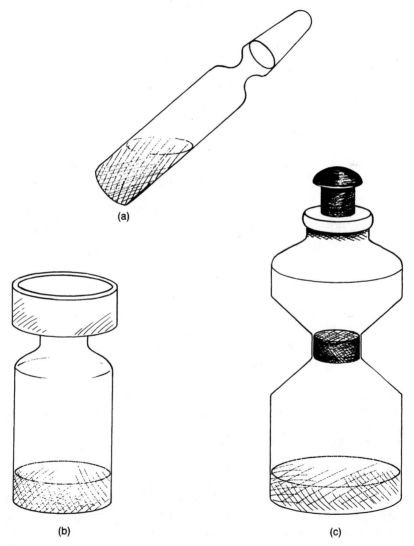

(a)

(b)

(c)

FIGURE 8.5. Packages for sterile powders. (a) Ampule; (b) vial with rubber
closure; (c) vial with two chambers.

the stopper in the rest of the way when the process is complete. A sterile powder and diluent can be packaged together in a vial with two separated chambers. Diluent in the upper chamber is combined with the powder in the lower chamber when pressure is applied via the top closure dislodging a rubber stopper between the two chambers [Figure 8.5(c)]. One example of this application is the packaging of vitamin B complex in the diluent and vitamin C as a sterile powder. This avoids the decomposition of vitamin C that is catalyzed by the decomposition products of vitamin B complex even in a dry mixture.

Tablets and Caplets

Tablets and caplets are packaged in glass or plastic bottles with screw caps or snap-on lids or in flexible structures. For ethical drugs, 60–70% of the packages are bottles; for OTC, 80% are in bottles. For both ethical and OTC drugs, 80–90% of the bottles used are plastic. Glass is still used where extreme product sensitivity to moisture or high product volatility demands the highest barrier or where package compatibility is an issue. However, nitroglycerin is the only instance in the USP listings for drugs in solid dosage forms where the preference for glass is specifically stated. One factor that diminishes the protection requirements for containers is the broad use of protective coatings for tablets. In several cases in the USP listings, coated tablets require only well-closed containers, while tight containers are specified for uncoated tablets; light-resistant needs are eliminated if opaque tablet coatings are used. The inclusion of desiccants allows plastic packages to be used for some moisture-sensitive products such as Bufferin and other buffered products.

HDPE dominates the plastic bottle market at 70% usage while the other plastics used, in order of decreasing frequency, are PVC, PET, PP, PETG and PS. HDPE is preferred because it is the least expensive way to provide the protection of tablets from moisture that is an almost universal need. Essential constituents for products such as vitamins and antibiotics often become inactivated by moisture. Aspirin may be hydrolyzed to release acetic and salicylic acids. Biologicals such as thyroid may putrify. Codeine becomes discolored. Disintegration time can be affected: disintegration times for prednisone tablets varied greatly on storage in different packages [7]. The appearance of sugar-coated tablets can be altered by moisture which reduces gloss and causes discoloration.

In the pharmacy, tablets are usually repackaged in the familiar amber PS or PP vial with a snap-on or CR screw cap. About 10% of the time, tablets are dispensed in their original containers. Drug companies offer smaller containers to encourage this practice.

A factor in the increasing use of plastics is their fabrication flexibility that is unmatched by glass or metal. Novel distinctive shapes are readily created. An example (Figure 8.2) is the new triangle-shaped Tums bottle where both bottle and cap have a flattened profile. The bottle is an injection-molded blend of PS and high-impact PS, and the cap is medium density PE [21].

On the other hand, the packager may want to use a plastic container that duplicates the appearance of glass. With this in mind, Senokot vegetable laxative tablets recently switched to injection blow molded PET bottles which are virtually identical to their glass predecessors and allow the brand to retain its identity. The switch to plastic was motivated by the desire for reduced weight and improved resistance to breakage [34].

Whether the container is glass or plastic, mechanical abrasion of tablets is a common problem during shipment and handling. This is avoided by filling the empty head space with (in the order of decreasing usage) cotton, rayon, polyurethane, or polyester fibers. However, the cottoning can be a source of moisture in the package. Even the so-called nonabsorbent grades of cotton may contain as much as 8% moisture and this is enough under the right temperature conditions to have an adverse effect on some products. For moisture sensitive drugs, the cotton must be dried before use or plastic materials should be used [35].

While unit dose packaging of solid oral dosage forms is growing it still accounts for only about 20% of OTC packages in the U.S. There is a higher usage of flexible packaging for ethical drugs largely for doctor's samples and hospitals. Although strip packaging was the first flexible package for tablets, blisters now dominate with an 80% share. For strip and blister packages, web composition is selected to provide the degree of product protection, the child resistance, and the presentation required. For blister packs the forming web is essentially always PVC (sometimes coated or laminated) and the lidding web can be paper/foil for push-through (which dominates in usage) or plastic or plastic/foil for access by peel. Peel access is preferred for fragile tablets.

A variation on the blister pack for OTC products is a thermo-formed tray, usually opaque, with each cavity holding a single tablet and covered with a peelable lidding film. One example, Romicol cough cubes, was described earlier. Another alternative for oral solids is the old standby, individual wrapping, to preserve freshness and provide easy portability for single units. Tempo, when introduced as a new, soft, chewable antacid cube, used a wax-coated paper/foil inner wrap on the cube and overwrapped five cubes into a pouch using a paper/ionomer/foil/ionomer structure. The roll or Life Saver package is occasionally used to provide ready portability for small quantities of, for example, antacid tablets.

For hospital dispensing, the traditional small cups of paper or PVC have been largely replaced by strip and blister packages with blisters dominating. Peel lidding is preferred for blister packs, with the lidding containing a paper layer so that all the necessary information accompanies every blister all the way to the nurse's station [25]. Recently a new aid for tablet dispensing was introduced: a zipper closure bag especially designed for containing blocks of blisters. Opaque areas on the bags allow for printing information on contents, dosage, patient name, etc., by the pharmacist [36].

In the early stages of this diversification of unit dose packages, concern was raised by the Drug Research and Testing Laboratory of the USP that hospital pharmacists needed more information on the barrier properties of the unit dose packages used for in-house packaging. A study made in 1977 of the packages being used in the Baltimore area showed that none provided good moisture barrier; the level of moisture pickup by desiccant pellets varied from 6 to 108 mg after storage for five days. The packages tested included PE bags, PVC cups with paper laminate covers, PE/cellophane-PE/foil strip packages and PVC-foil blisters. The blisters provided the best protection [37].

Since these early studies, the ability of blister packs to match the moisture protection of rigid containers has been well established. Not only did a recent study confirm this but it provided evidence also for an added advantage of blister packs over conventional multiple unit packages. A blister protects a moisture-sensitive tablet right up to administration whereas in a multiple unit bottle the moisture in the head space is continually replaced as the bottle is repeatedly opened. For ibuprofen tablets it was shown that the process of repeated opening and closing of a bottle can increase the moisture pickup by 20–35%, depending on tablet count, under severe storage conditions (78°F and 85% RH for six months). By using an ACLAR laminate blister construction, protection similar to that provided by an always-closed bottle was achieved [38].

Just as questions were raised about moisture barrier with the increasing use of flexible unit dose packages, so also were concerns about loss of potency for highly volatile products such as nitroglycerin tablets. Stabilizing additives are effective in reducing the vapor pressure of nitroglycerin so that loss by permeation is controllable. However, sorption remains a problem. When tablets were stored in conventional strip packages of aluminum foil laminated to LDPE film (film next to tablets), 90% loss in potency was found for unstabilized tablets.

One study included a variety of thermoplastic sealants for the strip packages [39]. These sealants included PVC, ionomers, and HDPE. Careful monitoring of nitroglycerin potency during storage revealed that sorption was a function of both the chemical structure and the crystallinity of the plastic layer. Thus the order of degree of sorption was PVC ≫ LDPE > ionomer > HDPE. The only structure which provided adequate retention of potency for two-year storage life was a foil lamination with ionomer as the seal layer. Another example of sorption occurred when uncoated aminophylline tablets (a smooth muscle relaxant used to treat bronchospasm) were packaged in clear cellophane sachets. The film discolored in three months and hospital pharmacists discarded the packages. The discoloration was found to be due to sorption of ethylenediamine released from the tablets [40].

Capsules

Bulk packaging of capsules is similar to that for tablets. Neither hard nor soft capsules require protection against mechanical shock. Soft capsules packaged in large quantities may deform and clump, particularly under warm conditions. Neither capsule requires much protection from moisture for reasonable storage periods, except in tropical climates where mold can be a problem.

Consumer and pharmacy packages are the same as for tablets for both multiple and single unit packaging. For soft capsules packages should have tight closures and plastics used should have good moisture barrier.

Suppositories

Suppositories (rectal, vaginal, and urethral) are made with fatty or glyco-gelatine bases so that the products are soft and will melt readily at body temperature. Therefore, for bulk packaging, quantities must be kept small (100–150) and placed in shallow boxes to minimize compression.

For consumer packaging, ten to twelve items are sometimes placed in greaseproofed cardboard boxes with means provided for separation of each item. Sometimes the items are individually wrapped with aluminum foil for aesthetic reasons. An alternative package consists of thermoformed PVC trays with five or six cavities. Two such trays are fitted top-to-top and heat sealed together. In another approach, the thermoformed cavities in a tray serve as molds in which the fluid formulation is allowed to solidify, allowing molding and packaging in one step. The top web is usually of foil or film and is adhered to the tray via an adhesive or heat seal layer. Sometimes, especially for exported products, the seal area is increased for added protection from moisture gain or ingredient loss. A major advantage of the formed tray is that if the item melts, its shape is reestablished upon cooling [41]. Some vaginal suppositories are molded tablets and are packaged like tablets.

PACKAGES FOR LIQUIDS

Liquids include oral, topical, and ophthalmic preparations.

Bulk Packaging

Plastic containers are mostly replacing glass for quantities of 10 gallons or less except where compatibility is an issue. A common plastic container is a brown tinted, one gallon HDPE jug. Large quantities of liquids are packaged in metal drums, often with liners, or fibreboard drums with blow molded PE inserts. Lids are usually steel or plastic.

Consumer and Pharmacy Packages

Oral Liquids

Multiple dose containers are either plastic or glass depending largely on compatibility and permeability considerations. Of all package types (premade bottles, pouches, form-fill-seal bottles, bags, prefilled syringes), 70–80% are premade bottles. The use frequency for the rest of the package forms is in descending order as listed. For bottles, plastics (largely HDPE) dominate. For OTC products, 80% or more of the bottles are plastic; the usage of plastic is lower for ethical drugs (about 50%) because of the greater potency and activity of these products [12].

Although HDPE is the dominant plastic with about 70% share, other plastics are also used for bottles. PVC has a higher barrier to oxygen, sulphur dioxide and alcohol than does HDPE. It will not stress crack in the presence of alcohol and has superior chemical resistance and better clarity. Early concerns about the possible leaching of additives from PVC led to numerous studies which showed fairly broad compatibility. In a typical study, test results were reported for a kaolin-pectin suspension in a sorbitol vehicle, cough syrup with a glucose syrup vehicle and B-complex elixir with an aqueous glycerin vehicle. All had retained a quality in PVC comparable to storage in glass. On the other hand, PVC containers were not suitable for an antibiotic suspension with chloramphenicol palmitate in sugar syrup with chloroform and other preservatives since this preparation curdled and discolored [42].

PET bottles are increasing in popularity because PET is readily recycled and closely resembles glass. For these reasons, Pepto-Bismol was recently introduced in a PET bottle with advertisements (*same shaped bottle . . . same quality product*) assuring consumers of no loss in protection [43]. PET is also used for Vicks Formula 44 liquid cough medicine. Here, an advantage cited is the consistency of the inner dimensions of the bottle which "assures not only uniform weights of the empty bottles but avoids the variation in fills which takes place when glass bottles vary in their inner dimensions, such as due to extra glass in the wall dimension" [44].

Plastic bottles are often preferred for the convenience features that can be added. Squeeze bottles for drops are often used for infant cold medications and analgesic products for relief of tooth and mouth pain. A more sophisticated application is the narcotic pain killer (morphine sulfate liquid) in a container designed to reduce the chance of under- or overdoses: an HDPE squeeze bottle equipped with a dip-tube device that dispenses a precisely metered dose for each squeeze [45]. This is a step beyond the more traditional approach of supplying a plastic cup with the bottle as is commonly done for liquid cold remedies.

While plastic bottles seem well entrenched for liquid products, the aseptic brick pack, which is commonly used in food packaging, is just finding its way into pharmaceuticals. In 1987 an oral rehydration solution, Resol, became the first U.S. application for this package. The product is used in the treatment of diarrhea, particularly in children. Although the package for the hospital version of the product is a glass bottle that can be fitted with a nipple, the brick pack was chosen for the one quart retail package because of the need for a sterile container that was attractive, not bulky, and easy to use. Plastic containers did not meet the needs for sterility and a two year shelf life. Metal cans were eliminated because of corrosion due to the high mineral content of the liquid [46].

In the unit dose packaging of oral liquids in hospitals, vials, cups and oral syringes are used broadly. Typical packages are one-half to one-ounce cups of aluminum or plastic laminations with a paper/foil lid adhered to the cup rim. Often these dosages are supplied prepackaged to the hospital. For in-house packaging one convenient system used is an amber plastic container which is supplied with a foil composite, peelable lid. It is filled through a hole in the bottom which is then plugged by forcing in an elastic ball. This approach avoids the need to develop the capability for applying the lidding in-house.

Some problems have been uncovered in the repackaging of oral liquids in single dose packages. Incompatibility with volatile flavor essences and the chemistry of the liquid drug itself have doomed some plastic cup laminations [47]. Special concerns have been raised about plastic oral syringes and a number of studies have been reported. For products with reasonable stability, plastic syringes offered satisfactory protection, only modestly inferior to glass vials, for storage at room temperature and below. As an example of such studies, cimetidine hydrochloride (for treatment of duodenal ulcers), furosemide (a diuretic), and theophyline (a bronchodilator) repackaged in PP oral syringes and glass vials all retained more than 90% potency after 180 days at 4° and 25°C [48].

Products that are inherently unstable exhibit relatively short shelf life in both plastic oral syringes and glass vials unless stored at low temperature. The superior protection of glass for these is pronounced at all temperatures. Typical of this kind of product are reconstituted penicillins. Penicillin V potassium in unit dose glass vials reached 90% of potency at room temperature in 5 days. Refrigerated storage extended the shelf life to about 30 days [49]. When stored in plastic syringes at 25°C, this same product reached 90% of labelled potency in less than 37 hours; with storage at 4°C 90% potency was retained for 11.5 days [50].

For retail consumer packages the use of unit dose for liquids is rare. Among the few examples to be found on drugstore shelves are PVC and PVC-laminate vials containing cough syrups and mouth rinses. These packages offer durability, ready portability and relative ease of opening [46]. A novel approach (see Figure 8.4) is premeasured unit doses of Robitussin cough medicine in blisters that are miniature versions of the regular Robitussin bottle. The bottle-shaped cavities are thermoformed from PVC laminated sheet and the top web is an aluminum foil laminate. The top of each blister has a snap-off, tamper evident dispensing feature for easy opening, and it can be squeezed for emptying. A two year shelf life is claimed for this package [51].

Topical Liquids

Multiple unit packages for skin preparations are primarily glass or plastic bottles. Various convenience dispensing systems are used to facilitate application of the product with minimum mess. Squeeze bottles with hinged tops for direct application of liquids to the skin and containers with mechanical pumps are often used. A recent introduction of an OTC acne medication features a HDPE bottle with a sponge-tip applicator activated by inverting the bottle and depressing the applicator to moisten the tip. Depressing the applicator opens the spring-loaded PP valve located below the sponge. The applicator housing is made of LDPE and a nylon cap screws on the top of the assembly [52].

Another common package for topical liquids, especially for low viscosity liquids applied as sprays and foams, is the aerosol container. Preparations for the treatment of dermatological conditions represent the largest application of this technology. These preparations are used as antipruritics or anti-inflammatory agents in the treatment of acne, poison ivy, and related conditions. Other applications of aerosols include local anesthetics for minor surgery (benzocaine, ethyl chloride, cyclomethylcaine, and tetracaine), muscle relaxants, analgesic preparations for relief of muscle and rheumatism pain, first aid and antiseptic sprays, antibiotic sprays, spray-on protective skin (collodion solution and sometimes including an antiseptic and anesthetic) and preparations for burn treatments. A recent innovation for burn treatment combines two containers to allow the creation of a cooling ice layer for the treatment of burns. One container is made of PE and has a mechanical spray pump which creates a water spray forming a layer of water on the affected area. The PE container is mounted on an aerosol can from which a spray is used in a second step to freeze the water into an ice layer [53].

For skin preparations, problems due to loss of ingredients and compatibility are not major factors in selecting packages, but some limitations have been encountered. For instance, some aqueous based lotions contain an organic solvent to increase ingredient solubility. This solvent can be lost by permeation as can phenolic substances used as disinfectants or bactericides. In oil/water emulsions, PP or PVC containers should be used to avoid stress cracking. For those oils which can permeate through plastic (especially LDPE), HDPE is preferred.

Beyond physicians' samples, there are few examples of unit dose packaging of skin preparations. Dosage control does not seem to be a significant need and portability is conveniently achieved using small multiple unit packages.

Ophthalmic Liquids

For ophthalmic liquids plastic squeeze bottles have almost completely replaced the traditional glass bottles with droppers. Since the plastic (usually LDPE) in these packages will not withstand autoclave temperatures, it is necessary to sterilize the container and fill it aseptically. Hospital pharmacists packaging experimental or specialty preparations generally use glass containers and sterilize by terminal autoclaving. Another limitation of the squeezable plastic container is compatibility. For example, LDPE can absorb bactericides used in the formulations. An unusual instance of leaching was uncovered in a study of the stability of an experimental ophthalmic solution in LDPE bottles. It was found that an ingredient from the adhesive used for the pressure sensitive labels was permeating through the PE container. As a result solutions became turbid and a blue deposit formed on the wall of the container. The concentration of the drug was not affected; the interaction was with the preservative, benzalkonium chloride [54].

Form-fill-seal systems are finding their way into the packaging of ophthalmic liquids. Sterility is assured by aseptic filling of the newly formed container while it is still hot. While both LDPE and PP are used, LDPE dominates with 85% share. The major advantage of the form-fill-seal approach is that empty bottles need not be shipped, stored and sterilized. This package is used for artificial tears [see Figure 8.6(a)]. The small packages offer ready portability and reduced tendency for contamination since each container supplies a limited number of drops. Advertising for this product emphasizes its freedom from preservatives [12].

Nasal and Bronchial Sprays and Inhalants

Broadly speaking, nasal and bronchial sprays and inhalants require that mists be created by the package. While, for nasal sprays, squeeze bottles have been the preferred package, recently several major OTC brands have switched to the metered pump [see Figure 8.6(b)], following a trend already underway in ethical products.

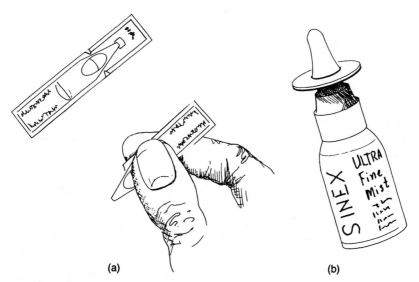

(a)   (b)

FIGURE 8.6. Packages for liquids. (a) Form-fill-seal package for artificial tears; (b) metered pump package for nasal spray.

The package features a valve system which delivers a precise dose of product when the consumer depresses the outer flange of the pump assembly. The metered pump has two advantages over the squeeze spray: dosage is more controlled and back suction of nasal discharge is prevented. A package with a pump is also used for Chloraseptic throat spray.

The most widely employed ingredient in nasal sprays is phenylephrine hydrochloride. Early studies were made to determine the possible loss of potency due to its sorption by a PE container. In one study no sorption of phenylephrine hydrochloride alone took place but, in conjunction with two different preservatives, binding of the active ingredient to the wall of the container occurred. This slight interaction was most significant at room temperature, with elevated temperature disrupting the apparent weak binding. Permeation of water through the container was also demonstrated but at a low rate which did not affect potency [15].

One form of bronchial medication is an inhalant which forms a vapor when added to hot water. Inhalants are packaged in bottles. A recent innovation that improves product safety and reduces consumer cost is a metered valve that dispenses Broncho Saline in 1 ml quantities from a pressurized metal container. This greatly facilitates the exact diluting of bronchodilator medications which are often prescribed for chronic lung conditions. Prediluted medications are much more costly [55].

The other form of bronchial medication is a mist created by the package. Aerosols with a convenient nozzle for directing the spray into the mouth and throat are the most common package. One example is shown in Figure 8.7(a). The container can also be fitted with a metered valve for precisely controlled dosage. While aerosols are used primarily for the treatment of nasal and bronchial conditions, they can also be used for systemic administration of drugs for other conditions provided the drug is capable of being deposited in the respiratory tract and is nonirritating. Examples of drugs now packaged as aerosols are epinephrine (for the emergency treatment of allergic reactions), isoproterenol (for treatment of congestive heart failure), octyl nitrite, phenylephrine, ergotamine (for treating vascular headaches), and dexamethasone (a steroid).

Up to this point, for these dosage forms, only multiple unit packages have been described. The few known examples of unit dose applications are for inhalants. Three ml quantities of Proven-

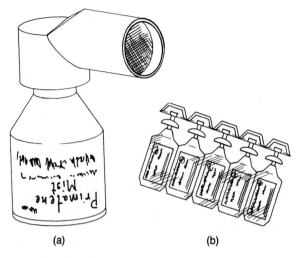

(a)   (b)

FIGURE 8.7. Examples of packages for bronchial mists and inhalants. (a) Aerosol package for bronchial mist; (b) form-fill-seal vials for respiratory therapeutic in brackets of five unit doses.

til bronchodilator are supplied in a HDPE bottle so that a single dose can be poured into an inhaler [56]. In a similar application, polyethylene vials produced on form-fill-seal machines are used for isoetharine respiratory therapeutic liquid. The vials are produced in brackets of five [Figure 8.7(b)] [57].

Enema Preparations

Formulated enema preparations are packaged as unit doses in convenient, squeezable plastic tubes that are extrusion blow molded, filled, and sealed aseptically [12].

Parenteral Preparations

Multidose packages for parenteral liquids are usually glass with elastomeric closures covered with metal or plastic caps. The container is either molded or made from glass tubing. The type of glass used depends on drug characteristics. Type I containers are suitable for all parenteral products. Type II containers are suitable for most large volume parenterals and some small volume parenterals. Type III containers are suitable for some nonaqueous products.

Many parenterals are susceptible to degradation initiated by absorption of light. Small volume parenteral packages present optimum conditions for photochemical and oxidative decomposition with their large ratio of surface area to formulation volume and ample unfilled headspace. Thus USP recommendations must be followed when packages are called for that are light-resistant and, in the most severe cases, that are opaque. The stability of parenterals can also be adversely affected by sterilization, so terminal sterilization is less common than aseptic filling of a sterilized vial [58].

As noted in Chapter Six a special concern for parenterals is drug loss through, and interaction with, the closures which must be made of an elastomer to allow multiple withdrawals of liquid without loss of sterility. The rubber closure "introduces a potential sink for volatile, lower molecular weight formulation components and a reservoir of potentially reactive extractables" [59]. Sorption of antimicrobial constituents is the most common problem. There are considerable variations among elastomeric compounds in the tendency for sorption, so that screening is important in selecting the best candidate. Teflon coated stoppers eliminate most sorption problems. Also, sufficient excess of the antimicrobials can usually be safely included in the formula to assure a reasonable shelf life. A less common problem is sorption of the drug itself by primary packaging components. Nitroglycerin is the most widely documented case. In one study, for example, it was shown that there was a 25% loss in nitroglycerin after 1000 hours even in glass ampules and almost 50% loss in vials with rubber stoppers in the same period. These authors speculated that the loss in the ampules could be due to sorption by an oil film on the glass which is almost impossible to remove even with repeated washings [60].

A special problem for vials with elastomeric closures is sprayback caused when drugs are reconstituted by inserting a needle and injecting diluent into the container. Since this can cause a positive pressure, a fine spray can be emitted when the needle is withdrawn. This is not a significant problem for most products but for injectable chemotherapy drugs it is desirable to reduce the introduction of these toxic products into the environment. A disposable top which snaps onto the vial is now available to contain any spray back [61].

A variety of packages, from glass ampules and vials to different types of syringes are used for parenterals in single dose form. Glass ampules have long been used since they provide the greatest assurance of retained sterility and drug potency during storage. However, they are inconvenient since the fused glass seal must be opened by breaking which can be dangerous to health personnel. An even greater disadvantage of the glass ampule is the potential for contamination of the injection with glass particles. While prescored ampules make opening somewhat safer, the contamination problem remains.

The extent of this problem is illustrated in one study where the mean number of particles found after opening single dose glass ampules was 14 from 1 ml ampules, 28 from 5 ml ampules and 32 from 20 ml ampules. Particle size, determined by light microscopy, ranged between 10 and 1000 microns [62]. The particle count would be much higher if the minimum detectable size had been lowered. In another study, electron microscopy was used to extend the range of observed particle size. For example, the number of glass particles introduced into a 5 g sample of a lyophilized semisynthesized penicillin, carbenicillin disodium, by opening a glass ampule became enormous (10^8 to 10^9) when the size limit was lowered to 0.1 millimicron [63]. This study showed that filter needles were ineffective in removing these particles. They apparently penetrated the filter under the force of aspiration. Small gauge needles were similarly ineffective. While little is known regarding the clinical significance of intravenous, epidural and subarachnoid injection of glass particles, there have been reports of pulmonary microemboli, thrombi, and granulomas as a result of small particle contamination found in large intravenous infusions [64]. In Japan, this problem is ameliorated by wrapping the ampule below and above the scored break-off line in two kinds of shrink film. The upper film sleeve is made to have high static charges which attract and hold glass particles produced by the breakage of the ampule.

Single dose vials with rubber closures are also used. Double-chambered vials are used to separately package components which are unstable when mixed (see Figure 8.4).

During World War II, the need for prefilled syringes for field use led to the development of a unit consisting of a flexible metal tube (like an ointment tube) fitted with a needle protected by a glass sleeve. A wire probe within the needle was used to puncture the tube. These units were used to package morphine sulfate. Problems with sterility, compatibility, and leakage limited broader adoption. Ampules fitted with needles were also an early but unsuccessful approach. A later and more successful approach, sterile prefilled syringes, offers ease of administration, reduction of errors and increased assurance of sterility. In most instances the injection is packaged in a glass cartridge with a needle attached and is administered by inserting the cartridge into a metal or plastic holder which may or may not be part of the original package. An example is shown in Figure 8.8(a). These packages are usually Type I glass for long-term stability. Often, the drug contacts the glass barrel, rubber closure, and stainless steel needle. However, some prefilled syringes limit the contact of the drug with the glass barrel and rubber component parts, and activation is required prior to injection.

A recently introduced innovation allows extensive process automation and lower cost along with the other advantages of prefilled syringes. Reminiscent of the WWII collapsible tube and needle combination, the liquid is encapsulated within a plastic bubble or blister in a form-fill-seal aseptic packaging operation. The

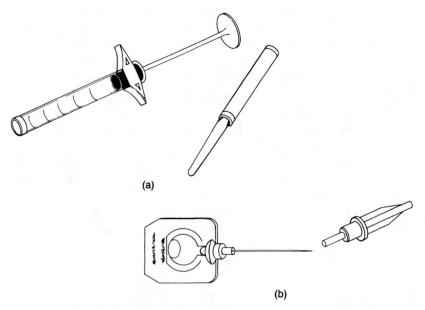

(a)

(b)

FIGURE 8.8. Unit dose packages for parenteral preparations. (a) Unit dose cartridge and needle with plastic holder; (b) form-fill-seal package for unit dose.

blister is then fitted with a needle and activator assembly. In use, the package is mechanically activated to permit flow into the needle and the liquid is expelled from the blister by squeezing [see Figure 8.8(b)] [65].

Drugs supplied in prefilled glass syringes include furosemide, diazepam (for management of anxiety), labetelol hydrochloride (for treatment of hypertension) and ketorolac tromethamine (a nonsteroidal anti-inflammatory) [66]. Another group of drugs supplied in prefilled syringes is used in cardiopulmonary resuscitation where the timely and accurate administration of emergency drugs (such as sodium bicarbonate, epinephrine, calcium chloride, lidocaine, isoproterenol, metaraminol and atropine) is critical.

Given the limited range of commercially available prefilled, disposable syringes, hospital pharmacies must do their own syringe prefilling for extemporaneous use and sometimes for storage. Often plastic syringes are used, but data on the effects of storing drugs in plastic syringes are limited and pharmacists therefore minimize storage or use freezers unless the specific drug of interest has been studied.

Interest in storing drugs in plastic syringes was shown as early as the late 1950s with data reported on the interaction of six bacteriostatic agents with nylon, PE, and PS syringes. Only nylon was found to bind these agents (47% to 85% loss) after one week at 30°C [67]. Sorption of sorbic acid by nylon was also reported and related to hydrogen bonding [68]. Since then studies have been reported of various drugs stored in plastic syringes. A summary is given in Table 8.4.

Paraldehyde was found by several investigators to be chemically altered when stored in plastic syringes. Gentamicin sulfate, an antibiotic, was found to lose an unacceptable amount of potency (>15%) after thirty days storage [71].

To determine how well plastic syringes protected drugs from microbial contamination from the environment, filled syringes were subjected to in-use conditions and intentional microbial challenge. It was concluded that plastic syringes apparently pose no additional contamination potential over glass [72].

Long term storage of frozen syringes has also been investigated for specific drugs. For example, carbenicillin and oxacillin (semi-synthesized penicillins) frozen in glass and plastic syringes remain stable after three months [73]. A group of antibiotics and

Table 8.4. Drugs stored satisfactorily in plastic syringes [69,70].

Drug	Use	Storage Time
Insulin	Treat diabetes	7 days*
Heparin	Anticoagulant	4 weeks
Hydroxyzine HCl	Manage anxiety	10 days
Atropine Sulfate	Emergency heart	10 days
Meperidine HCl	Narcotic analgesic	10 days
Tobramycin	Antibiotic	2 months
5-Fluorouracil	Treat various carcinomas	7 days
Thiamine HCl	Nutritional supplement	84 days
Cytarabine	Treat leukemia	7 days
Doxorubicin HCl	Treat leukemia	5 days
Methotrexate Na	Treat leukemia, carcinomas	30 days
Chlorpromazine HCl	Treat psychotic disorders	1 year
Sodium Bicarbonate		3 months*

*Refrigerated; remainder at room temperature.

penicillins (cephalothin, cefazolin, cefamandole, and nafcillin) can all be used after nine months frozen storage in glass syringes [74]. Frozen plastic syringes were judged also to be comparable to glass in protecting drugs from microbial contamination [75].

In summary, it must be emphasized that despite numerous studies, generalities are both difficult and dangerous. The general feeling is that those wishing to store drugs in syringes, especially in plastic, need to determine to their own satisfaction the suitability of such a practice.

While systems for prefilling syringes with liquids have been available for some time, it is only recently that prefill glass syringes have been available for freeze-dried injectables that can be reconstituted within the syringe. One type of two-chambered syringe is depicted in Figure 8.9(a). When the cap is depressed, the glass plunger/container is pressed inward, displacing the liquid diluent just enough to force the stopper, which separates the chambers, into a larger diameter section of the plunger/container [Figure 8.9(b)]. The solid and liquid are then mixed by shaking. Next, rear and front caps are removed and the plunger is depressed further so that the larger diameter section reaches a rubber valve which expands, providing an opening for the reconstituted fluid to flow through a canal to the needle [Figure 8.9(c)]. In another type of two-chambered syringe, the separation plug is designed so that the diluent is swirled by a vortex as it enters the chamber with the solid drug to enhance dissolution. In both types the drug is freeze-dried in the syringe and then the plug and diluent are added [76,77].

IV Fluids

Intravenous fluids are packaged in containers that have closures which can be penetrated by needles or spikes to gain access to the fluid. Containers for IV fluids must be designed to maintain solution sterility and be free of particulate matter and pyrogens through storage and administration. Various types of packages for IV fluids are depicted in Figure 8.10 [78]. To facilitate hanging,

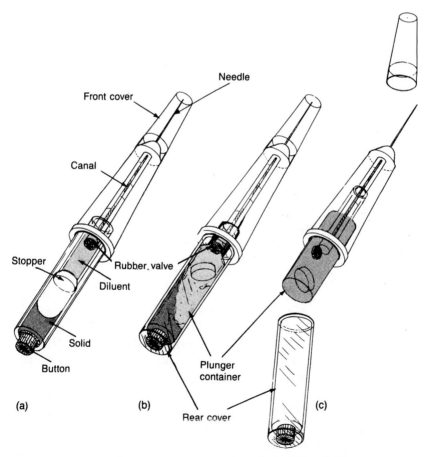

FIGURE 8.9. Two compartment syringe for solid and diluent.

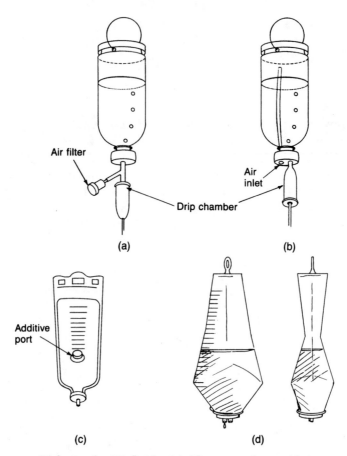

FIGURE 8.10. Packages for IV fluids. (a) Glass container with vent and air filter; (b) glass container with vent tube; (c) flexible plastic bag; (d) semi-rigid plastic container: front and side views.

glass containers are fitted with aluminum or plastic bands; plastic containers are fabricated with eyelets or straps. The fluid is transported from the container to the point of injection through administration sets consisting of a plastic spike to pierce the closure, a drip chamber to trap air and provide a visual indication of flow rate, and a length of PVC tubing.

Containers are either glass or plastic; the latter may be either rigid or flexible. For the rigid containers, plastic is rapidly displacing glass because of greater safety, lighter weight, lower cost and generally greater convenience. Use of plastic also eliminates concerns about alkali extracted from glass—a common problem with electrolytes. Reduced particulate contamination is also an advantage claimed for plastic. Particulate matter is especially critical for IV fluids because of the large volumes administered intravenously.

The plastic used for rigid containers is almost always PP with some HDPE, rigid PVC, or copolyester also used. Coextruded high barrier plastic containers have been popular for some time in food packaging. A similar container using EVOH as the barrier layer was recently announced for enteral feeding liquids [79]. Another innovation for plastic containers is the blow-fill-seal process where aseptic filling is coupled with package formation using a semirigid PE container.

Flexible plastic containers for IV fluids have important advantages over rigid containers. As fluid leaves a rigid container, air must flow in to fill the emptied volume. Some arrangements for venting are shown in Figure 8.10. This requirement does not apply to flexible containers which collapse as fluid is withdrawn. This also means that auxiliary microbial air filters on the vents are not necessary for flexible containers thus reducing cost, complexity and uncertainty. Intermediate in performance are PE semirigid containers which collapse to some extent but not enough to totally eliminate the need to introduce replacement air. For the flexible bag, ease of disposal is another plus. Also the bags can be squeezed by a pressure cuff (pressure infusion) for rapid emergency administration of large quantities of liquids.

Plastic IV packages have some disadvantages. All IV containers have visible scales to allow the delivered volume to be monitored. Plastic containers are less transparent than glass, which makes the determination of liquid level and inspection for turbidity more difficult. As usual with plastic there are concerns about potency changes caused by sorption and permeability, and contamination due to leaching. These concerns are amplified for IV fluids because of the relatively high volumes administered.

Standard IV fluids such as those containing dextrose, electrolytes and/or amino acids are available prepackaged as are some stable drug solutions including ranitidine HCl, simetadine, theophylline and gentamycin. Where it is necessary to make up IV mixtures in the pharmacy, drugs are injected into a bag prepackaged with diluent. Where a mixture requires many components (e.g., for total parenteral nutrition), computerized systems can be used to automatically pump controlled amounts of liquids from a number of reservoirs into an IV bag. Such a system provides ready monitoring of the amount of each liquid that is added [80].

Often, instead of using an IV mixture that is purchased or prepared in the pharmacy, a drug is added piggyback-style using the primary IV fluid as a vehicle to administer another drug. Administration sets allow such an introduction either by a syringe or from a separate container designed for ready connection to a second administration set that joins the primary set using a Y-connector. This separate container is often a 250 ml bottle or bag which is partially filled with a vehicle such as saline solution. The drug, which is reconstituted first as necessary in its parenteral vial, is then added to the piggyback package using a syringe. Alternatively, some drugs are supplied as prepackaged fluids which can be directly connected to the administration set thus reducing hospital labor and the risks of errors.

Some of these prepackaged systems are specifically designed to minimize drug loss due to rapid chemical change in unstable mixtures. These losses are reported to be 6–9% in the best hospitals and much higher in others [81]. In one such system, an adaptation of the traditional piggyback technique, antibiotic powders that are unstable when mixed with water (Kefzol, Mandol, and ampicillin) are supplied in a plastic container to which an appropriate diluent is introduced using a syringe. Newer systems eliminate the need for secondary administration sets and provide an even more convenient and foolproof means of handling unstable admixtures. In Baxter's system, unstable mixtures are delivered frozen in PVC bags to be stored in a freezer until use. An advantage of the frozen system is that no manipulation to achieve mixing is required. In Abbott's Add-Vantage system, a plastic bag is partially filled with diluent and the drug is in a separate glass vial encased in a plastic cover. The user removes the cover, locks the vial onto a chamber on top of the bag and mixes the drug into the solution by external manipulation of the stopper on the vial (see Figure 8.11). The adoption of this new system was rapid, with over forty different drugs packaged this way only one year after introduction in 1985. It is claimed that this system reduces hospital time and labor by 60% and drug wastage by 20%. Hospitals tend to use either one or the other of these last two systems [80].

For two incompatible fluids, a convenient IV fluid package is

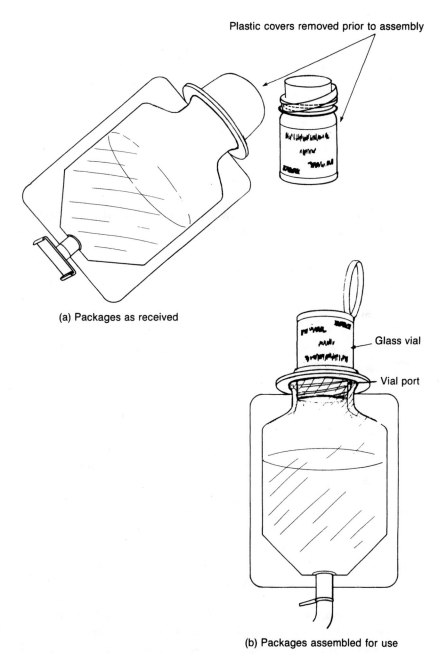

Plastic covers removed prior to assembly

(a) Packages as received

Glass vial

Vial port

(b) Packages assembled for use

FIGURE 8.11. Package for convenient, sterile mixing of IV fluid with additives.

the Nutrimix container. Here two separate solutions are contained in one bag compartmentalized by a clamp. It is used to separately package dextrose and amino acid solutions which are not compatible. The clamp is removed at bedside allowing mixing just prior to administration. In this case, a different plastic, a copolyester elastomer, had to be used for the bag since PVC tends to seal to itself under the pressure of the clamp [81].

Increasing use is being made of home IV therapy for pain management, chemotherapy, antibiotic therapy, etc. Numerous portable infusion devices are commercially available. One example is the CADD-PCA infusion pump to which a medication cassette containing the IV formulation is attached. These cassettes can be filled in the pharmacy according to prescription [82].

With the increasing use of plastic packages for IV fluids, extensive compatibility studies have been made. These studies focused on PVC bags. Wang and Chien list sixty-eight drugs for which results on sorption in PVC bags were reported in the period of the mid-1960s to the early 1980s [14]. In twelve cases significant losses in potency were reported over storage periods ranging from eight hours to one week. These drugs were chlormethiazole edisylate, diethylstilbestrol diphosphate disodium (a synthetic estrogen), isosorbide dinitrate (for treating angina pectoris), a group of drugs for treating anxiety disorders (diazepam, medazepam, nitrazepam, and oxazepam), metholhexital sodium (an anesthetic), nitroglycerin, retinol acetate, thiopental sodium and warfarin sodium (an anticoagulant). Insulin, nitroglycerin and diazepam have been studied extensively.

Since insulin is not lipophilic, absorption into plastics is theoretically unlikely. Indeed, some studies showed the loss of potency to be about equal for glass or plastic, suggesting surface adsorption only [83–86]. Furthermore, the addition of small amounts of several substances, including human serum albumin, polygelin, and human blood, have been reported to be effective in minimizing drug loss [83,87,88].

Nitroglycerin, on the other hand, has a strong affinity for PVC and the sorption process has been analyzed quantitatively by several workers leading to models that adequately describe it [39,89–92]. Most studies have reported much higher losses in PVC bags versus glass bottles although the situation is confused somewhat by reports of sorption of nitroglycerin to be essentially the same for glass and plastic [93–96]. Finally, one study showed very little loss of potency in PE containers [97]. The upshot of these extensive investigations is the following recommendations: "Hard solid plastics such as polyethylene and polypropylene generally do not absorb nitroglycerin. Consequently, it is recommended that only infusion solution containers made from glass or a plastic known to be compatible with nitroglycerin (i.e., polyolefin) be used . . ." [98].

For diazepam, large losses of potency have been clearly identified with absorption in PVC bags [99,100]. Therefore, the recommendation again is to use only polyolefin or glass containers.

In addition to sorption, leaching of possible toxic constituents is a special concern for PVC bags which contain large amounts of plasticizers. Several workers have identified the presence of these plasticizers in blood and plasma stored in PVC bags. In turn, the presence of plasticizer in the tissues of patients receiving blood transfusions has also been established [101,102]. Similarly, plasticizers in IV fluids from PVC have been identified [103]. Because plasticizers are insoluble in water, they can appear as globules [104,105]. As might be expected, the presence of alcohol increases the amount of plasticizer leached from PVC. Edible oils used in total nutrition systems also enhance leaching [106–108].

Permeation of water through PVC bags can lead to a significant change in solution concentration during long-term storage of standard IV fluids. Weight losses of water in PVC bags in ambient conditions for eighty-four days have been reported to be 14%, 9%, and 4% for volumes of 50, 100, and 500 ml respectively [109]. The use of higher barrier overwraps essentially eliminates this concern.

Despite these concerns about PVC bags, they continue to be widely used since many IV mixtures are sufficiently compatible with the bag, and storage of drugs in PVC bags is often limited to the period of administration. It is critical, however, that evaluations of specific drug mixtures are carried out under the conditions intended for storage and use of the PVC bag. Looking to the future, efforts which have been underway for some time to find a suitable alternative material are bearing fruit.

A commercial product has been introduced: a multilayer bag whose principal layer is an E/P random copolymer. As might be expected with the conservatism that necessarily surrounds IV fluids, adoptions of this new bag are slow. Nevertheless, continuing evolution of plastics and multilayer film technology makes likely the eventual success in producing an IV bag that performs as well as PVC without its deficiencies.

PACKAGES FOR SEMISOLIDS

Semisolids include ointments, creams, and pastes for ophthalmic and topical applications.

Bulk Packages

Large quantities of semisolids are packaged in stainless steel, mild steel, or tinplate drums. Plastic liners are used where appropriate. Plastic containers such as HDPE buckets with a snap-on lid are also common, but are less suitable for ointments with high water content and long storage.

Medium bulk quantities are packaged in jars and tins. When glass jars are used, amber glass is preferable since many preparations — for example those containing phenolic compounds — are light sensitive and change color. Plastic jars are usually of PS or PP. Anhydrous ointments devoid of reactive ingredients can be packaged in tins but lacquering is required for aqueous preparations. Lanolin causes rusting of even lacquered metal and is supplied in plastic or glass. Phenolic or mercurial salts also lead to corrosion.

Consumer and Pharmacy Packages

Collapsible tubes have become the most popular package for most semisolids because of convenience and better protection from contamination when the product is withdrawn. In fact, collapsible tubes are obligatory for sterile preparations. Plastic tubes dominate over metal with the breakdown being about 50% PE, 40% plastic-laminated, and 10% aluminum [12]. While collapsible metal tubes offer good protection from product oxidation and desiccation, the tubes crack and leak, labels tend to disintegrate after many uses, and there are compatibility limitations. Corrosive ointments, such as buffered ointments, attack steel tubes though aluminum tubes or internal lacquers generally solve the problem.

Polyethylene tubes are lower cost, hold their shape, and preserve graphics better than labels glued to metal tubes. Plastic eliminates metal particles sometimes found in metal tubes which are a serious problem for ophthalmic ointments. A problem with plastic tubes is the lack of deadfold which leads to shape recovery that causes suck-back of air, desiccation, and oxidation. There are also, of course, the usual concerns about permeability and absorption. Aseptic packaging rather than terminal sterilization is required for plastic tubes.

Plastic laminate tubes are more flexible than either aluminum or PE and less liable to material failure on repeated use or as a result of attack by the product. They are completely resistant to essential oils, air, odors, and light. The potential for multicolor artwork is greater on laminate tubes. Because of these advantages, laminate tubes are increasingly used in pharmaceuticals, especially for OTC products. A recent list, shown in Table 8.5, illustrates the variety of topical preparations now in laminated tubes [110].

Another advantage for tubes over jars is that convenience features can be readily added. One example is a metered dose cap which is used for Retin-A, a topical acne preparation, that assures just the right dosage each time for maximum effectiveness [111].

Jars, when used, are of glass or plastic and although PE, PS, PVC and PP are all used, there are some limitations. Both PVC and PS are attacked by methyl salicylate. Dimethyl phthalate and other phthalate esters attack polystyrene, and fixed oils lead to stress cracking in PS.

Table 8.5. *Topical preparations packaged in plastic laminate tubes.*

Acne preparations	Dry skin treatments
Analgesic creams	First aid ointments
Antibiotic ointments	Hemorrhoid preparations
Antifungal creams and ointments	Herpes treatments
Anti-itch creams and ointments	Jock itch treatments
Athlete's foot preparations	Mucous membrane anesthetics
Breast creams	Muscle deep-heating rubs
Burn preparations	Topical antibacterial agents
Cortisone ointments and creams	Vaginal creams
Dermatoses treatments	Zinc oxide creams
Diaper rash preventatives	

A new package for semisolids is the toothpaste pump. This package was introduced for Myoflex analgesic creme which is also offered in large jars and HDPE tubes. The pump is designed for users, especially those with arthritis, who have difficulty opening other containers. An easily removed cover provides access to the creme by the simple pressure of one finger. Since the valve cleanly cuts away the ribbon of the product, there is no product withdrawal back into the container, as with conventional tubes. Product in this higher cost package is sold at a 10% premium [112].

Single dose packages such as pouches or sachets offer the advantages of superior convenience and contamination prevention but are as yet too costly for consumer use.

PACKAGES FOR TRANSDERMAL SYSTEMS

Transdermal patches are packaged in individual pouches and less often in thermoformed trays. Since these products often contain volatile ingredients, film structures with a high barrier layer (aluminum foil, metallized film or PVDC coating) are usually employed. The seal layer is typically LDPE. The bulk package is a carton and pharmacists repackage the product generally into small boxes.

SUMMARY

This overview of the packaging of the various dosage forms has focused on current practice with emphasis on trends in package choices and new innovations. Clearly, at the leading edge of change are plastic packages, single dose offerings and a host of convenience features. The driving forces for the adoption of these changes are rooted in the determinants discussed in the first part of this chapter with the strongest (for OTC) being product differentiation. As more and more ethical drugs are switched to OTC, drug packagers will increasingly use the newer packaging technologies.

The descriptions of packaging problems for the various dosage forms are based largely on published information which in turn is dominated by studies on injectable products where the consequences of package interactions and failures are the most severe. The literature consists of studies by hospital pharmacists and academic personnel. Very little information on packaging problems is available from drug manufacturers that could provide insight into package development problems and market failures. Thus this chapter reflects an outsider's view.

Nevertheless, it seems apparent that there have been no catastrophic packaging problems such as product spoilage, significant loss in potency before the expiration date or gross leakage from package breakdown. The absence of such catastrophic packaging problems is largely a result of the very conservative environment within the drug industry and the FDA and the maturity of packaging materials technology: the limitations of materials can be readily anticipated. For plastics in particular, drug manufacturers benefit from the longer history of use in food packaging.

Lest these considerations breed complacency, it should be pointed out that nearly 3000 packaging problems that could have led to product adulteration were reported during the period 1982–1987 [113]. Furthermore, potency losses or product contamination due to package incompatibility are impossible for the consumer to detect. Thus, the caution that each drug must be tested in its actual package cannot be overemphasized.

REFERENCES

1. 1989. "General Notices," *USP XXII*, p. 8.
2. *USP XXII*, p. 1575.
3. *USP XXII*, p. 1570.
4. *USP XXII*, p. 1576.
5. *USP XXII*, p. 1575.
6. Rabinow, B., R. Payton and N. Raghavan. 1986. *J. Pharm Sci.*, 75:808.
7. David, S. T. and C. E. Gallian. 1986. *Drug Dev. and Ind. Pharm.*, 12:2541–2550.
8. Taborsky-Urdinola, C. J., V. A. Gray and L. T. Grady. 1981. *Am. J. Hosp. Pharm.*, 38:1322–1326.
9. *USP XXII*, p. 1574.
10. Wang, J. Y. and Y. W. Chien. 1984. *Sterile Pharmaceutical Pack-*

aging: *Compatibility and Stability.* Philadelphia, PA: Parenteral Drug Association, Inc., pp. 107–125.

11. Brennan, A. 1991. *TAPPI Proceedings: Polymers, Laminations & Coatings Conference,* pp. 473–479.
12. T. Williams, PACO Corporation, private communication, 1991.
13. "General Notices," *USP XXII,* p. 8.
14. Wang and Chien, pp. 51–56.
15. Karig, A., E. P. Garnet and G. J. Sperandio. 1973. *J. Pharm. Sci.,* 62:396–402.
16. Wang and Chien, p. 49.
17. *USP XXII,* pp. 1571–1572.
18. *USP XXII,* pp. 1495–1500.
19. Cafmeyer, N. R. and B. B. Wolfson. 1991. *Am. J. Hosp. Pharm.,* 48:736.
20. Gerstman, R. 1984. *Pharmaceutical Executive* (February): 34–40.
21. Knill, B. J. 1989. *Food & Drug Pkg.* (March):3.
22. Anon. 1990. *Packaging Digest* (August):74.
23. O'Brien, R. 1990. *Food & Drug Pkg.* (March):3.
24. Anon. 1991. *Chain Drug Review* (January):1.
25. O'Brien, R. 1990. *Food & Drug Pkg.* (April):4.
26. D. Kanemori, ICI Pharmaceuticals, private communication, 1991.
27. Mullen, J. C. 1990. Presentation to *Pharmaceutical Symposium, Puerto Rico, February 16, 1990.*
28. Anon. 1990. *Food & Drug Pkg.* (September):31.
29. Ericson, G. 1989. *Packaging* (April):481–490.
30. Reiterer, F. 1991. *Pharmaceutical Technology* (March):74–80.
31. Anon. 1985. *Packaging* (May):13.
32. Anon. 1987. *Manufacturing Chemist* (August):29.
33. Pesko, L. J. 1991. *American Druggist* (March):80.
34. Anon. 1991. *Pkg. Digest* (May):20.
35. Ross, C. F. 1983. *Packaging of Pharmaceuticals.* Leicestershire, U.K.: The Institute of Packaging, p. 5.
36. Anon. 1991. *Pkg. Digest* (September):112.
37. Reamer, J. T., L. T. Grady, R. F. Shangraw and A. M. Mehta. 1977. *Am. J. Hosp. Pharm.,* 34:35–42.

38. Pires, C. L., J. R. Giacin and H. E. Lackhart. 1988. *J. Pkg. Technology*, 2:213–217.
39. Pikal, M. J., D. A. Bibler and B. Rutherford. 1977. *J. Pharm. Sci.*, 66:1293–1297.
40. Estabrook, D. R., D. J. Stennett and J. W. Ayres. 1980. *Am. J. Hosp. Pharm.*, 37:1046.
41. Ross, C. F., pp. 7–8.
42. Shah, R. C., P. V. Raman and B. M. Shah. 1978. *Pharm. J.* (July 15):58–59.
43. 1990. *Packaging Digest* (June).
44. Holmgren, B. R. 1985. *Pkg.*, pp. 46–50.
45. Forcinio, H. 1988. *Food and Drug Pkg.* (December):31.
46. Anon. 1987. *Packaging Digest* (May):58–59.
47. Larson, M. 1991. *Packaging* (January):30–32.
48. Christensen, J. M., R.-Y. Lee and K. A. Parrott. 1983. *Am. J. Hosp. Pharm.*, 40:612–615.
49. Allen, L. V., Jr. and P. Lo. 1979. *Am. J. Hosp. Pharm.*, 36:209–211.
50. Grogan, L. J., B. K. Jensen, M. C. Makoid and J. N. Baldwin. 1979. *Am. J. Hosp. Pharm.*, 36:205–208.
51. Anon. 1991. *Packaging Digest* (May):78–79.
52. Anon. 1991. *Food and Drug Packaging* (July):4.
53. Anon. 1989. *Food and Drug Packaging* (December):20.
54. Chrai, S., S. Gupta and K. Brychta. 1977. *Bull Parenteral Drug Assoc.*, 31:195–200.
55. Anon. 1991. *Packaging*, p. 21.
56. Anon. 1991. *Packaging Digest* (May):38–40.
57. Anon. 1987. *Packaging* (April):87.
58. B. Smith, West Corporation, private communication, 1991.
59. Mendenhall, D. W. 1984. *Drg. Dev. and Ind. Pharm.*, 10:1297–1342.
60. Sturek, J. K., T. D. Sokoloski, W. T. Winsley and P. E. Stach. 1978. *Am. J. Hosp. Pharm.*, 35:537–540.
61. Anon. 1990. *Packaging* (April):18.
62. Carbone-Traber, K. B. and C. A. Shanks. 1986. *Anesth. Analg.*, 65:1361–1363.
63. Bollinger, R. O., A. M. Preuss, P. R. McClain and W. T. Hill, Jr. 1978. *Am. J. Hosp. Pharm.*, 35:312–316.

64. Waller, D. G. and C. F. George. 1986. *Br. Med. J.*, 292:714.

65. 1991. UniJect System Product Literature, Acacia Laboratories, Santa Ana, CA.

66. 1991. *Physicians' Desk Reference*. Oradell, NJ: Medical Economics Data, pp. 403–438.

67. Marcus, E., H. K. Kim and J. Autian. 1959. *J. Am. Pharm. Assoc.*, 48:457.

68. Rodell, M. B., W. L. Guess and J. Autian. 1964. *J. Pharm. Sci.*, 53:873.

69. Turco, S. and R. E. King. 1987. *Sterile Dosage Forms. Their Preparation and Clinical Application*. Philadelphia, PA: Lea and Febiger, pp. 276–277.

70. Hicks, C. I., J. P. B. Gallardo and J. K. Guillory. 1972. *Am. J. Hosp. Pharm.*, 29:210–216.

71. Weiner, B., D. J. McNeely, R. M. Kluge and R. B. Stewart. 1976. *Am. Soc. Hosp. Pharm.*, 33:1254–1259.

72. Huey, W. Y. 1985. *Am. J. Hosp. Pharm.*, 43:78.

73. Kressel, J. J. 1978. *Am. J. Hosp. Pharm.*, 35:310.

74. Kleinberg, M. L., G. L. Stauffer, R. B. Prior and C. J. Latiolais. 1980. *Am. J. Hosp. Pharm.*, 37:1087–1088.

75. Mitrano, F. P. 1986. *Am. J. Hosp. Pharm.*, 43:78.

76. 1991. Preject (R) product literature, Preject Inc., Warwick, RI.

77. Watts, J. 1988. *Manufacturing Chemist*, 59:31,33.

78. Gennaro, A. R., ed. 1990. *Remington's Pharmaceutical Sciences, 18th Edition*. Easton, PA: Mack Publishing Company, pp. 1572–1575.

79. Anon. 1988. *Packaging Digest* (August):55.

80. Bourret, J., director, Dept. of Pharmacy Services, Hospital of the University of Pennsylvania, private communication, 1991.

81. Russo, J. R. 1986. *Packaging* (February):26–32.

82. Allen, K. V. 1990. *U.S. Pharm.* (March):72–74.

83. Kraegen, E. W., L. Lasarus, H. Meler, L. Campbell and Y. O. Chia. 1981. *Br. Med. J.*, 3:464.

84. Weber, S. S., W. A. Wood and E. A. Jackson. 1977. *Am. J. Hosp. Pharm.*, 34:353.

85. Whalen, F. J., W. K. Lecain and J. Clifton. 1979. *Am. J. Hosp. Pharm.*, 36:330.

86. Okamoto, H., T. Kikuchi and H. Tanizawa. 1979. *Yakuzaigaku*, 39:407.

87. Weisenfeld, S., S. Podolsky, M. D. Goldsmith and L. Ziff. 1968. *Diabetes*, 17:766.

88. Kerchner, J., D. M. Colaluca and R. P. Juhl. 1980. *Am. J. Hosp. Pharm.*, 37:1323.

89. Roberts, M. S., A. E. Polack, G. Martin and H. D. Blackburn. 1979. *Int. J. Pharm.*, 2:295.

90. Roberts, M. S., P. A. Cossum, A. J. Galbraith and G. W. Boyd. 1980. *J. Pharm. Pharmacol.*, 32:237.

91. Illum, L. and H. Bundgaard. 1982. *Int. J. Pharm.*, 10:339.

92. Malick, A. W., A. H. Amann, D. M. Baaske and R. G. Stolle. 1981. *J. Pharm. Sci.*, 70:798.

93. Cossum, P. A., M. S. Roberts, A. J. Galbraith and G. W. Boyd. 1978. *Lancet*, 2:349.

94. Crouthemel, W. G., B. Dorsch and R. Sahangraw. 1978. *N. Engl. J. Med.*, 293:262.

95. Boylan, J. C., R. I. Robison and P. M. Terrill. 1978. *Am. J. Hosp. Pharm.*, 35:1031.

96. Ludwig, D. J. and C. T. Ueda. 1978. *Am. J. Hosp. Pharm.*, 35:541.

97. Yliruusi, J. K., A. G. Sothmann, R. H. Laine, R. A. Rajasilta and E. R. Kristoffersson. 1982. *Am. J. Hosp. Pharm.*, 39:1018.

98. Trissel, L. A. 1990. *Handbook on Injectable Drugs, 6th Edition*, ASHP, p. 56.

99. Mackichan, J., P. K. Duffner and M. E. Cohen. 1979. *N. Engl. J. Med.*, 301:332.

100. Parker, W. A., M. E. Morris and C. M. Shearer. 1979. *Am. J. Hosp. Pharm.*, 36:505.

101. Gesler, R. M. and N. J. Kartinos. 1970. *Lancet*, p. 151.

102. Jaeger, R. J. and R. J. Rubin. 1970. *Science*, 170:460.

103. Moorhatch, P. and W. L. Chiou. 1974. *Am. J. Hosp. Pharm.*, 31:149.

104. Whitlow, R. J., T. E. Needham and L. A. Luzzi. 1974. *J. Pharm. Sci.*, 63:1610.

105. Needham, T. E. and L. A. Luzzi. 1973. *N. Engl. J. Med.*, 202:1256.

106. Corley, J. H., T. E. Needham, E. D. Sumner and R. Mikeal. 1977. *Am. J. Hosp. Pharm.*, 34:259.

107. Kampouris, E. M. 1976. *Polymer Eng. Sci.*, 16:59.

108. Kampouris, E. M., R. Regas, S. Rokatas, S. Polychronakis and M. Pantazoglou. 1976. *Polymer*, 16:840.

109. Stauffer, G. L., M. L. Kleinberg, K. R. Rogers and C. J. Latiolais. 1981. *Am. J. Hosp. Pharm.*, 38:998.

110. K. Rawden, American National Can Company, private communication, 1991.

111. Anon. 1990. *Packaging* (June):9.

112. Anon. 1987. *Packaging Digest* (May):34–35.

113. Hamilton, R. E. 1988. "Adulteration of Drugs and Drug Products," *Encyclopedia of Pharmaceutical Technology, Vol. 1.* New York, NY: Marcel Dekker, p. 188.

GENERAL REFERENCES

Gennaro, A. R., ed. 1990. *Remington's Pharmaceutical Sciences, 18th Edition.* Easton, PA: Mack Publishing Co.

King, R. E. 1984. *Dispensing of Medication, Ninth Edition.* Easton, PA: Mack Publishing Co.

Lachman, L., H. A. Lieberman and J. L. Kanig. 1986. *The Theory and Practice of Industrial Pharmacy, Second Edition.* Philadelphia, PA: Lea and Febiger.

Ross, C. F. 1983. *Packaging of Pharmaceuticals.* Leicestershire, U.K.: The Institute of Packaging.

Turco, S. and R. E. King. 1974. *Sterile Dosage Forms.* Philadelphia, PA: Lea and Febiger.

Wang, Y. J. and Y. W. Chien. 1984. *Sterile Pharmaceutical Packaging: Compatibility and Stability.* Philadelphia, PA: Parenteral Drug Association, Inc.

CHAPTER NINE

Issues in Modern Drug Packaging

In addition to the basic and ever-present requirements of product protection and low cost, five major issues confront those who are responsible for packaging drugs in the U.S. today:

- harmonizing child resistant closure requirements with the need to make the contents of drug packages more readily accessible to the elderly
- improving tamper evident features and discovering better ways of alerting customers to those features
- increasing the frequency of unit dose packaging in situations where it is economically justified
- improving patient compliance through innovative package design
- dealing with the "green packaging" movement with its antiplastic overtones that oppose the trend to replace glass and metals with plastics

The first two issues, both related to closures, were treated in Chapter Six. This chapter will cover the remaining three.

UNIT DOSE PACKAGING

As noted earlier, a unit dose package is one which contains the particular dose of the nonparenteral drug prescribed or ordered by the physician for the patient. This package may or may not be the same as a package that only contains one unit, since the dose prescribed may be more than one unit.

The discussion of this subject will be divided into two sections:

one devoted to unit dose packaging in and for hospitals and one devoted to unit dose packaging for the retail pharmacy. The distinction between unit dose and a package that contains only one unit differs in importance for these two market segments. In hospitals that have adopted the unit dose packaging and delivery system, all packages of nonparenterals that go to the patient are unit dose packages. In the retail pharmacy, where no repackaging takes place, those few drugs that are individually packaged are done so with only one unit in the package, since it is impractical for the manufacturer to anticipate prescriptions that call for more than one drug unit to be taken at a time. Thus some are unit dose packages and some are not.

Unit dose packaging for the pharmacy has become an issue in pharmaceutical packaging because today there is conflict between drug manufacturers, who prefer to package most drugs in multiple unit packages, and those who believe that consumers would be better served by unit dose packages. So far, the manufacturers are winning the battle. As discussed below, the frequency of unit dose packaging for retail drugs is relatively low.

Unit Dose Packaging in Hospitals

In hospitals, recent ASHP studies show that unit dose dispensing systems have largely replaced the traditional practice of dispensing pills or liquids out of stock bottles into little paper cups for delivery to the patient's bedside [1]. Whether done by the nurse from a stock bottle or by the pharmacist, the possibility for error in that traditional system is so high that patient safety has been the major driving force for unit dose packaging, where each tablet or liquid dose can be clearly identified as to identity and strength and coupled with the patient's name.

There is no longer any real debate about the advantages of unit dose packaging for dispensing of drugs in hospitals. Although the advantages have been cited many times in publications over the past thirty years, the following summary prepared by ASHP may be the most comprehensive [2]:

- The frequency of medication errors is reduced.
- The total cost of the drug dispensing system is reduced.
- Pharmacist and nurse time can be increasingly devoted to patient care activities.

- Overall drug control is improved and drug use can be more effectively monitored.
- Patient billings for drugs are more accurate.
- The pharmacist(s) has/have greater control over pharmacy workloads and staffing.
- Drug inventories in patient-care areas are greatly reduced.
- Computerization and automation are facilitated, bringing improvements in efficiency and accuracy.
- Unused medications can be safely recycled into stock for reuse.

This long list of benefits has led ASHP to take the official position that ". . . the unit dose system . . . [is] an essential part of drug distribution and control in hospitals . . ." [2]. To further reinforce this position, two states, New York and New Jersey, now require that hospitals in those states dispense all drugs to inpatients in unit dose form.

The 1990 ASHP survey of short term, nonfederal hospitals revealed that a complete unit dose system is now offered by 89% of the responding hospitals, compared to 74% in 1987 and 18% in 1975 [1]. Furthermore, there is essentially no size-related bias in the figures—unit dose systems are used as frequently in small hospitals as in large ones.

To achieve these impressive results, four problem areas had to be confronted and solved in each hospital:

- Unit dose dispensing requires additional space, both for packaged drug storage and for the in-house packaging equipment that is required.
- Dosages differ and depend on the patient's situation and the approach of the individual physician.
- Many of the unit doses required are not packaged by drug manufacturers.
- The cost of drugs packaged by the manufacturer as single units is higher than the cost of those same drugs packaged in the 500-count bottle that would be the normal order size for a large hospital pharmacy.

Satisfactory resolution of these problems and complete implementation of a unit dose distribution system in a hospital requires that the hospital pharmacy install drug repackaging equipment, since no drug manufacturer can be expected to anticipate the entire variety of physician prescriptions. This is the one major disadvantage of unit dose dispensing in hospitals: everyone recognizes that a manufacturer can do a better packaging job than can a hospital pharmacist.

To a degree, the hospital repackaging operation has been supplanted by drug repackagers who supply the packages that hospitals want, but there are limits to this arrangement as well: repackagers can practically handle only drug units for which there is a predictable and steady demand; and if drug stability is at risk when packaged in single unit form, it is better to do the repackaging near the time of use and in the hospital rather than have it done by a separate repackaging company. Nitroglycerin, with its well-known stability problems, is the most extreme example of this latter problem — it is never repackaged commercially.

The dosage forms that are most frequently repackaged are oral solids and oral liquids. Oral liquids lag behind oral solids, but most observers predict a boom in liquid medications [3]. For one example, liquids have become crucial in medicating elderly patients who have trouble swallowing. However, packaging liquids in unit dose form is difficult, because of the potential for leakage and interaction with the container. As noted in Chapter Eight, the most common liquid package is the one-half to one-ounce plastic cup lidded with peelable foil that carries the necessary printed information. These cups are assembled in tens or dozens in shrink wrapped trays. Blister packaging may eventually replace this system.

Injectable liquids can be, and also are, repackaged in single dose form, but the more stringent sterility requirements for these products represent an additional challenge and an additional motivation for the hospital to purchase these prepackaged where possible.

Recognizing that most hospital pharmacists have accepted the need for in-house repackaging, manufacturers of drug packaging machinery have developed systems which can turn this necessity into an advantage: automated packaging machines that store hundreds of different solid dosage forms in separate bins which feed a strip packaging line. When the menu of drugs that is wanted for, say, the next eight hours is entered into the machine's computer, it automatically feeds the right tablets or capsules into the packaging line where they are individually packaged between two strips of LDPE heat sealed around the dose and labeled typically with drug identity, dose, lot number, expiration date and patient's name. The sequence in which the items are packaged can be determined either by administration time or by medication type. The label can include a bar code for use in cases where the patient's wristband is also bar coded; in this way the nurse equipped with a portable scanner can further confirm that the dose to be given the patient matches the dose prescribed.

The major benefit offered by the manufacturers of these machines is reduction in cost. Not only is labor saved, but of comparable importance is the opportunity for the hospital to buy drugs in bulk and reduce its dependence on a repackager. Use of these machines conflicts with the desires of those who wish to see unit dose packaging more widespread on the retail scene. As manufacturers see their demand for unit dose packaging in hospitals decline, any incentive to offer the same packaging to their retail customers also declines.

To assist the hospital pharmacist in unit dose repackaging operations, ASHP has issued a *Technical Assistance Bulletin* which spells out guidelines on such matters as [4]:

- isolation of the operation
- number of products packaged at the same time
- handling finished packages, unused stock and unused labels
- inspection of stock and packages before beginning a packaging run
- necessary data that should be collected on packaging materials
- record keeping, monitoring and control
- how the expiration date should be determined
- storage procedures for repackaged products

Unit Dose Packaging for Retail Drug Distribution

The situation and the issues surrounding dispensing of drugs in unit dose form in the retail environment are starkly different from hospital dispensing. In contrast to the roughly 90% of hospitals that have adopted unit dose dispensing, only about 20% of all solid oral dosage forms are packaged as single units for OTC and retail pharmacy dispensing, and almost no liquid oral dosage forms are packaged as single units for this market. Recalling that the hospital market for drugs is about 10% of the total drug market in the U.S., we see that the overall frequency of unit dose packaging and dispensing is only a little greater than 20%. This low figure is all the more remarkable when compared to the situation in Europe—there, over 90% of prescription and OTC drugs dispensed at retail are packaged as single units.

The difference between European practice and U.S. practice has led to much speculation as to cause, and to a major organized effort by a group of packaging companies and manufacturers of flexible packaging materials, all of whom have a financial stake in increasing the frequency of blister packaging, to increase the use of the blister package for solid oral dosage forms.

Advocates of blister packaging cite four arguments in its favor: improved compliance, lower possibility of accidental misuse including but not limited to greater child safety, better product protection, and better tamper evidence. Of these, the first two receive major emphasis, while the last two arguments are less persuasive. Tamper evidence can be achieved in many alternative ways, as can product protection, although studies cited in Chapter Eight have shown that a bottle of moisture-sensitive tablets, if reopened and reclosed many times, will ultimately offer less protection than is afforded by a blister package.

The safety argument rests on the undeniable fact that the blister or strip package is the only one that yields only one tablet when it is opened. Many studies have shown that other forms of child-resistant packages are subverted by the user, either by repackaging the drug in a non-child-resistant container or by not properly securing the child-resistant closure. The other side of the coin, however, was detailed in Chapter Seven—children in test panels typically open from three to five blisters. If three to five tablets constitute a dose harmful to a 25-pound child, that blister package fails the child-resistant test. Thus the safety aspects of unit dose packaging in blisters are ambiguous unless the packaged drug offers little toxicity potential or unless blister designs are carefully chosen with the needs of both child safety and adult convenience kept in mind.

None of these child protection vs. blister design issues are important in Europe, where it is assumed, evidently without proof, that if a blister is opaque, children won't be sufficiently interested to open it. This is the first of several reasons why blister packages are more prevalent in Europe.

The compliance argument deserves close attention, since it is a major problem in U.S. healthcare today. Some key statistics illustrate this point.

- Almost 50% of the 1.8 billion prescription medications dispensed annually are not taken correctly by patients [6].
- About 125,000 Americans die each year because they fail to take medications as prescribed [6].
- One researcher [7] has estimated that only one-third of all patients take all their prescribed medicine, while one-third take only some, and an astonishing one-third take none at all!
- In Oregon, nearly 10% of all hospital admissions have been reported to be the result of pharmaceutical noncompliance.
- The U.S. Chamber of Commerce estimated in 1984 that noncompliance caused a $13–15 billion loss to the economy due to increased use of medical resources, unnecessary physician visits, therapeutic failure and prolonged illness [8].

The article by Dorothy Smith quoted in Reference [6] contains an excellent example that makes the case in a convincing way: the official labeling for Questran (cholestyramine), a drug administered to control blood plasma cholesterol levels, cites tests showing that full compliance with the recommended dose regimen lowered the incidence of coronary heart disease by 39.3%. However, since only about 50% of the participants in the clinical trial were fully compliant, the average risk among all the participants was lowered by only 19% [9].

Noncompliance is a long-standing problem. Journal articles that are now almost twenty years old list many studies that had been conducted before then to expose the situation and to urge corrective measures.

The problem is particularly acute among older people, with forgetfulness and the need to take multiple types of medication being the major causes of their noncompliance [10]. It will worsen as the population ages and as the elderly continue to be a disproportionately large consumer of prescription drugs.

Of the five major reasons for noncompliance that have been reported by the National Council for Patient Information and Education, three are related to the drug package and could be favorably influenced by packaging designed to increase compliance:

- taking an incorrect dose
- forgetting to take a dose
- taking a dose at the wrong time

It is widely agreed that improved patient education, which can take many forms, is needed to reduce the scope of this problem. Packaging that is designed to improve compliance is but one tool in this educational effort, but it may be the most important, since it is likely to be not only lowest cost but also the approach that continues to remind and urge the patient to comply, something that the physician and the pharmacist can do only once [11].

The occasional need for the patient to take more than one medication at a time can lead to confusion and exacerbate the noncompliance problem. This part of the problem would disappear if the combination of medications needed could be packaged together — several in one blister, for example. In some states, this is against the law, so USP, in an effort to promote this practice, formally recognized what they call *patient med paks*, provided guidelines for their use, and stated that the pharmacist may provide such a package with the consent of the patient and the physician [12].

Drug packagers have created a variety of compliance designs, all based on the unit dose principle. Empty packages, called *Mediset* or *Dosette*, which have separate dated pill slots for a weekly supply, can be purchased and filled by the patient, the nurse, the physician, or the pharmacist. Several early studies showed impressive gains in compliance when the Mediset was used [13]. Nevertheless, this device has never caught on in a major way, with cost, availability, ignorance, and apathy probably being the major reasons. Arguably, it is an extreme case of repackaging which should not be necessary.

There are a few examples of manufacturer's unit dose packaging of prescription drugs that have improved compliance:

- Lilly has provided nizatidine in a *Convenience-Pak* that reminds duodenal ulcer patients to take a tablet every evening.
- Norwich Eaton has packaged Macrodantin (nitrofurantoin) antibiotic in a so-called *MACPAC* which consists of seven blister pack cards, each containing four doses labeled with the time of day. Each card can be easily carried around (as

a bottle cannot). Included between Day 2 and Day 3 is a reminder card which urges the patient to take all the prescribed doses and explains why that is necessary.

- Allergan Pharmaceuticals provides a special cap, called a *C Cap Compliance Cap*, to fit their line of glaucoma medications. The cap has numbered stations that are revealed in sequence when the cap is rotated. After taking the medication, the patient rotates the cap to the new number as a reminder that the next medication will be the second, for example, of the day. These caps can also be provided with days of the week for medications to be taken once daily. This is a particularly interesting case of compliance packaging, since it deals with an asymptomatic situation—one where there are no disease symptoms to remind the patient to take the medication. A study showed that compliance improved from 55% to 84% when these caps were used [14]. Other closure manufacturers are offering closures containing mechanisms which advance a clock or other timekeeping device each time the medication is taken [15].

- Prescription vials containing microelectronic medication monitors in the cap have been developed and are useful in clinical trials with ambulatory patients because they record each time the vial is opened. Such devices are far too expensive for routine use, but could be the forerunners of devices that might someday be widely used as compliance aids.

- Perhaps the best known manufacturer's package is the *Dialpak* for contraceptive pills which consists of a molded plastic disc that rotates over another plastic disc containing cavities holding one pill each. The entire array is dated so there can be no doubt whether or not the pill was taken. Given the enormous emotional, social, and financial consequences of unwanted pregnancies, the high cost of this package is easy to justify, but for most prescription drugs, many of which must be taken even after the symptoms and thus the motivation disappear, a lower cost approach must be used if packaging is to have a significant impact on the compliance problem.

More complex and expensive devices have been developed to

improve compliance. Typical of these is the *Medi-Monitor*, a small battery-powered device that holds a day's supply of medicine (which may be of more than one type) that beeps to alert the patient when to take each medication and warns the patient against taking the wrong medication. Not yet commercially available, this device is unlikely to find widespread application because of its high cost [16].

Today's technology offers the unit dose blister package as the lowest cost way to provide a package that will increase compliance. For example, calendar blister packs have emerged as the most widely used packaging format for prescription drugs dispensed by nursing homes. If the patient notes on the strip of blisters the date administration began, inspection of the number of remaining doses and a knowledge of the present date leads to the conclusion that another dose is due. Addition of features such as printing the days of the week on the package can provide an additional assist, but there may not be room for such adornment— the case for widespread use of unit dose packaging in blisters must rest on the efficacy of the lower-cost unprinted package [17].

Several studies have suggested that unit dose packaging in blisters does improve compliance, but more data may be needed to create an overwhelmingly convincing case [18]. The Healthcare Compliance Packaging Council plans such studies, but a word of caution is in order. It would be a grievous mistake to assume that packaging alone can solve the problem. A very important cause of noncompliance is the deliberate, conscious decision by the patient not to follow the physician's advice. One study showed that 14% of prescriptions are never filled [19]. Another study showed that 21% of patients have at least once chosen not to follow their physician's advice. The most common reason was that they did not think the prescribed medication would be beneficial, but other reasons were fear of side effects or the fact that the symptoms had disappeared [20].

Another argument frequently made to support more widespread use of unit dose packaging is the *pharmacist time* argument—the training and experience of the pharmacist is used most effectively when it is devoted to patient counseling rather than to drug packaging. While it is difficult to argue with this generality, it is unlikely that an argument of this kind will have much impact on the situation that now exists in the U.S.

A major question that still remains is why unit dose packaging of prescription and OTC drugs is the exception in the U.S. while being the rule in Europe. So many reasons can be marshalled to explain why unit dose blister packaging is *not* dominant in the U.S. that it seems as if the question should be reversed, i.e., why is blister packaging so prevalent in Europe?

There are five constituencies that impact the degree to which unit dose blister packaging, as opposed to bulk packaging in bottles, is used for oral solid dosage forms: drug manufacturers; drug prescribers; pharmacists and drug chain managers; and the patient, or drug consumer.

The Drug Consumer

The average buyer of prescription or OTC drugs knows nothing about the issues of unit dose packaging or compliance. Thus the buyer puts no pressure on the immediate supplier—the pharmacist. It should be noted, however, that in areas where drugs in blister packs are more common than in the U.S., consumers generally favor this packaging method, finding it clean, safe and convenient from the portability standpoint [21]. Thus if blister packaging ever becomes widespread in the U.S., consumer preference will help it remain dominant.

The Pharmacist

The retail pharmacist may be one of the major obstacles to the widespread adoption of unit dose blister packaging. While we have not conducted a broad survey of pharmacists, some interviews and discussions with other industry experts reveal at least three reasons for pharmacists' lack of enthusiasm for unit dose packaging:

- If the pharmacist fills a prescription by removing a large blister pack card from a drawer, tears off the right number of individual doses, puts on a label and hands the result to the patient in a bag, his major occupation and the historical foundation of his profession have both been compromised, even trivialized. Historically, pharmacists have always compounded prescriptions. In the early days, the pharmacist actually combined various ingredients. Today, of course, most solid dosage forms are compounded by the drug companies, but some of the early pharmacist's function still lingers in the act of removing tablets from a large bottle and repackaging them in a smaller bottle. The argument that unit dose packaging will free up the pharmacist for more patient consulting probably does not carry much weight with most pharmacists who are usually shielded from the patient by a rack of merchandise and a clerk who passes out the filled prescriptions and collects the money.

- Blister packaging creates a space problem in the average pharmacy, or at least that is the perception of most pharmacists.
- Many pharmacists believe that blister packaging will be more expensive than bottle packaging. As we shall see, they have good reason for this belief. Naturally, they fear that they will be unable to recover this added cost from their customers.

The owners and managers of drug chains have a somewhat different view: they are beginning to favor unit dose packaging because they see it as a way to make their pharmacies more efficient. Filling a prescription by tearing off the right number of blister packaged pills is faster than counting out the correct number of pills and then repackaging that amount. Further, since the blister packed array does not require another container, the cost of the familiar, amber colored vial can be saved, helping to offset the higher cost of the blister package.

Over time, pharmacist resistance may become increasingly irrelevant as patent expirations move more drugs to generic status. Multiple source drug availability will foster the increased use of packaging as a selling tool, thus favoring the blister package that is preferred by many consumers [22].

Healthcare Providers

Physicians interpose a minor barrier to unit dose packaging in the U.S., when compared to their European counterparts. In Europe, prescription orders are usually worded *small*, *medium*, or *large*, referring to the three sizes of blister packs that have been adopted by European manufacturers. In the U.S., prescriptions are written by number, and the number usually does not match a standard blister pack count. Although this seems like a minor barrier, it is real—pharmacists do not want the undispensed tag ends of blister packs that they would have to dispense to some indifferent customer or try to return to the drug company for credit and repackaging.

The Drug Companies

The drug companies probably see more negatives in unit dose blister packaging than the other constituencies discussed above.

Conversion to blister packaging requires them either to make new investment and to obsolete depreciated investment, thus adding to cost, or to use contract packagers, also a higher cost alternative.

Accurate cost figures on blister packaging vs. bottle packaging are not available. The Healthcare Compliance Packaging Council plans such a study. The best figures available at this time suggest that blister packaging is cheaper for small package counts in the 50 to 100 range, and more expensive for package counts greater than 100 [23]. More tablets and capsules are packaged by drug companies in containers holding 100 or more items than in smaller containers. There are at least two reasons for this. First, hospitals and retail pharmacists buy in larger quantities to save money. Second, some consumer sizes of prescription drugs are large because the drug itself is taken for long periods of time rather than to cure a specific ailment. Antihypertensives are one example, thyroid supplements another. If rough estimates that show that the blister–bottle cost crossover is below 100 count are borne out by a more careful study, switching to blister packaging will increase packaging costs substantially.

As for any package change, FDA approval would be required, a process costing time and money.

Since prescriptions are not standardized, there is no single number that represents a unit dose for any drug. Some prescriptions call for "two every four hours," some for "one every four hours," etc. The only way the packager can manage this problem is to package single units. If a unit dose is really two units, single unit packaging adds to costs and the storage space dilemma.

Most customers, other than hospitals, are not pushing the drug companies to switch to unit dose blister packaging; some customers may even be opposed to the idea.

And finally, many elderly-friendly and traditional blister designs will not pass the child-resistant test if the drug is toxic to children in small doses.

It appears that this last factor is in part responsible for the large difference in frequency of blister package use in the U.S. as opposed to Europe. The child-resistant closure regulations in Europe, where they exist at all, are far less stringent than in the U.S. Another reason for the Europe-U.S. difference lies in differences in the health plans in the two areas. In Europe, most health plans limit the number of units that can be prescribed at one time to a ten-day to two-week supply. In the U.S., insurers will tolerate a longer supply period—thirty to sixty days. The smaller European purchase quantity favors blister packaging with its lower cost for packaging small numbers of items.

In summary, it appears that the future of retail unit dose blister packaging in the U.S. will be determined by the twin issues of compliance and cost. If non-blister package designs that increase compliance become more prevalent, and if a persuasive case cannot be made for blister packaging being of lower cost for packages as large as 100 count, the use of blisters will not increase far beyond the present level. Of these two issues, cost will ultimately prove to be the most influential determinant.

GREEN PACKAGING

This term has been widely adopted in recent years to denote packaging and packaging practices which are environmentally friendly. All packagers of goods are impacted to some degree by the current environmental attitudes; packagers of drugs are no exception. Since environmental pressures on packaging will become more severe as time passes, a brief review of this subject is warranted.

The environmental problem has its origins in the municipal waste disposal practices that were adopted many years ago by most American communities. The seemingly endless expanses of land available to Americans made the practice of land dumping, later upgraded cosmetically to landfilling, the most expeditious and least expensive way to dispose of municipal garbage and trash. So long as the landfill was remote enough to be unobtrusive, there was no problem.

Increasing population in the high population states along the Eastern seaboard and the emerging awareness that these landfills were in some cases contaminating aquifers used for drinking water has led to increased regulation of the landfilling process, to the closing of some landfills, and to the increasing scarcity of land available to expand this trash disposal process. These factors in turn have led in recent years to sharp escalation of waste disposal costs in some municipalities. This cost increase quickly got the attention of a formerly indifferent public who promptly pressured their elected officials to take action.

Concurrently, in the 1970s the EPA saw this as a situation requiring their intervention. The agency financed several studies that quantified the problem and developed the outlines of a plan to deal with it. This plan established a hierarchy of solutions, beginning with the most desirable and ending with the least desirable.

Source Reduction

The most desirable solution is called *source reduction*, which in layman's terms means, "use less, discard less, save more, reuse more." When applied to packaging, the source reduction approach attempts to reduce the volume and the weight of packaging materials and to eliminate packages which are not essential to the protection of package contents. A box containing a bottle is one classic example of the latter. Since no packager spends money needlessly, it is evident that all package elements perform some function that the packager regards as important. The problem is that functions considered important by packagers are sometimes considered wasteful and unnecessary by segments of the consuming public who are concerned about the environmental impact of packaging waste. Thus packagers, including those who package drugs, are now scrutinizing their packages more carefully to see if some elements can be eliminated and if the total weight and volume of package components can be reduced without compromising the safety and efficacy of their products.

Recycling

The next most desirable solution is recycling. Valuable packaging materials such as aluminum have been extensively recycled for years. More recently, paper and glass have joined the list of recyclable packaging materials, as have a few plastics. Recycling will undoubtedly become more widespread in the future partly because local laws will require it and partly because influential sections of the public feel that it's a good idea. This will happen even though the economics of recycling are dubious in many cases.

A side effect of the recycling movement is the pressure on package designers and packaging material manufacturers to make packages, particularly plastic packages, more recyclable. This will impact the multilayer plastic package that is widely used to package food, but is unlikely to have a measurable impact on drug packagers who rarely use these complex structures. It will also impact the choice of plastics as materials for containers. Until the plastics industry establishes a recycling infrastructure that convinces the public that all the major packaging plastics are not only recyclable but being recycled, the plastics that are not seen as being recycled are in danger of tax penalties or even outright bans. Right now, the race is on to set up recycling systems that will avoid either of these unattractive outcomes. So far, this situation has not had any discernible effect on the choices of plastic packaging materials made by the drug companies.

Incineration

The third most desirable solution is incineration, for which a more elegant term is *waste-to-energy conversion*. Incineration is a tough sell in many communities, since it requires a multimillion dollar installation that no one wants in his or her backyard. Nevertheless, incineration and sale of the byproduct energy are expected by the EPA to partly replace landfilling in the future.

One consequence of this trend will be pressure to diminish the amount of chlorine-containing plastics in the incinerator feed. Although well designed and well operated incinerators can safely handle the chlorine-containing byproducts of incinerated PVC and PVDC, many people are incorrectly convinced that increased dioxin levels will be an inevitable consequence of burning PVC. This belief is negatively impacting PVC packaging in some European countries. So far, European restrictions have been focused on food packaging. Drug manufacturers there have resisted substituting another material for PVC in blister packages because the properties of PVC make it well suited to this application. U.S. drug packagers' concerns about PVC will continue to focus on possible harmful effects of plasticizers and other additives (see Chapter Four); the incineration problem *per se* will have little impact on the use of PVC in drug packages.

Landfilling and Degradability

Landfilling is the least desirable of the options on the EPA's list, but it will continue to be the major waste disposal method for many years to come. The current public belief is that plastics, and plastic packages in particular, are the major cause of the landfill problem. The numbers clearly show this is not true. Widely publicized studies by Franklin Associates show that plastics *of all kinds* constitute only 7% by weight and 18% by volume of municipal trash. It is true that plastic waste will not degrade in a landfill, but it is also true that in a dry landfill, very few materials decompose [24]. Nevertheless, this misconception about degradability has led to public pressure and some legislative initiatives that advocate the development and use of degradable plastics. Degradable plastics, whatever their other merits, are not likely to find any application in drug packaging where long term package integrity is supremely important.

The same misconception about degradability also leads to pressure to switch packages from plastics to other materials that are believed to be more recyclable than plastics (such as glass) or more degradable than plastics (such as paper). We believe most drug packagers will remain immune to these pressures. The package is too important to the total drug product to be altered by ill-informed pressures of this kind which in any case are mainly directed not at drugs but at packages for food (e.g., the McDonald's clamshell decision) and other consumer goods where alternative materials are sometimes a more feasible option.

Summary

In summary, drug packagers, all aware of the green packaging movement and its growing importance, are generally doing what they can prudently do, such as source reduction, to help with the problem but they are not letting the environmental situation dictate their packaging decisions.

REFERENCES

1. Crawford, S. Y. 1990. *Am. J. Hosp. Pharm.*, 47:2665.
2. Anon. 1981. *Am. J. Hosp. Pharm.*, 38:1214.
3. Larson, M. 1992. *Proceedings of Conference on Pharmaceutical Packaging Outlook '92*, Avalon Communications, P.O. Box 505, Southampton, PA 18966.
4. Anon. 1983. *Am. J. Hosp. Pharm.*, 40:451.
5. Smith, D. L. 1989. *Am. Pharm.*, NS29:42.
6. Anon. 1987. *Schering Report IX: The Forgetful Patient: The High Cost of Patient Compliance.*
7. Haynes. 1989. *NCPIE Prescription Monthly.*
8. Kuperberg, J. R., et al. 1989. *Pharm. Exec.*
9. Anon. 1984. *J. Am. Med. Assn.*, 251:351.
10. Strandberg, L. R. 1984. *Am. Health Care Assn. J.*, 10:20; Erickson, G. 1990. *Packaging*, p. 58; Smith, D. L., op. cit., p. 42.
11. Rudd, P. 1979. *Clin. Pharm. Therapeutics*, 25:257.
12. *USP XXII*, p. 1574.
13. Anon. 1977. *Hosp. Pharm.*, 12:301.
14. Kramer. 1987. *Invest. Ophthalmol. Vis. Sci.*, 28:377.
15. Anon. 1989. *Food & Drug Packaging* (July):28.
16. Anon. 1991. *Drug Topics* (February 4):31.
17. Gerald Frank, Rorer Pharmaceuticals, private communication, 1992.
18. Wong. 1987. *J. Am. Geriatrics Soc.* (January):35.
19. 1985. *National Prescription Buyer's Survey*, The Upjohn Co., Kalamazoo, MI.
20. 1984. *Prescription Drugs: A Survey of Consumer Use*. Washington, D.C.: AARP.
21. Roberts, K. 1988. *Pharm. J.* (March 19):382.
22. Martineau, W. D. 1992. *Proceedings of Conference on Pharmaceutical Packaging Outlook '92*, Avalon Communications, P.O. Box 505, Southampton, PA 18966.
23. Erickson, G. 1989. *Packaging* (April):97; Mullen, J. C. 1990. *Puerto Rico Packaging Symposium*, February 16; Knud Christiansen, Klockner-Pentaplast, and Daniel Gerner, Packaging Coordinators, Inc., private communications, 1992.
24. Rathge, W. L. 1989. *Atlantic Monthly* (December):99.

GLOSSARY

A

absorption—The assimilation of one substance by another in a process which involves the diffusion of the substance being absorbed into the absorbing substrate.

acid—A chemical compound containing a hydrogen atom that, in water, dissociates from the molecule as a hydronium ion.

ACLAR—The Allied-Signal tradename for polymerized chloro-trifluoroethylene.

activator—In an aerosol container, the device that both releases the contents when the valve is pressed by the user and determines the character of the mist by the design of the orifice and expansion chambers.

administration—The passage of a drug into the body. The routes of administration may be oral, otic, ophthalmic, rectal, vaginal, subcutaneous, etc.

adsorption—The attachment of one substance (*adsorbate*) onto the surface of another (*adsorbent*) by means of a strong interaction between the two substances. Differs from *absorption* in that the two substances are joined only at the surface of the adsorbent, whereas absorption involves the penetration of the absorbate into the absorbent.

aerosol—A dispersion of submicron-size liquid droplets or solid particles in a gas. Used in packaging as a label for all liquid or semisolid products dispensed under pressure.

Al_2O_3—Aluminum oxide.

alkali, alkaline—Alkaline refers to aqueous solutions whose pH is greater than seven. An *alkali* is any substance, usually a metal oxide or hydroxide, that produces this condition when dissolved in water.

amide—An organic compound containing an $>N-C=O$ group.

amine—An organic derivative of ammonia.

amorphous—Without structure, not crystalline. When used in plastics technology, *amorphous* refers to a domain in a plastic that consists of molecules packed in a random fashion.

ampule—A piece of glass tubing, sealed at both ends, that contains a quantity of a drug intended for injection into the body.

analgesic—A substance that relieves pain.

anesthetic—A drug that abolishes or suppresses sensations such as pain by affecting either the central nervous system (general anesthetic) or peripheral nerve structures (local anesthetic).

angina—Any inflammatory disease of the throat or fauces. Often used as synonymous with angina pectoris, a heart disease characterized by intermittent chest pain coupled with feelings of suffocation.

angstrom (Å)—A unit of length equal to one-hundred-millionth of a centimeter.

antibiotics—Substances that inhibit the growth of or destroy microorganisms.

antihistamines—Substances that neutralize or inhibit the effects of histamine released in the body during allergic reactions.

anti-inflammatories—Substances that inhibit inflammation of tissue.

antimicrobial—Refers to substances that destroy microorganisms.

antioxidants—Compounds that react with oxygen. When blended into an oxidizable substance such as a plastic, antioxidants will react preferentially with oxygen and prevent oxidation of the plastic.

antipruritic—A substance that relieves itching.

antiseptic—A substance that inhibits the growth of microorganisms.

aseptic filling—The process of combining sterilized pharmaceuticals with sterile packages in a sterile environment.

ASHP—American Society of Hospital Pharmacists.

assay—The determination of the concentration of the active ingredient in a pharmaceutical.

ASTM—American Society for Testing Materials.

astringent—A substance that contracts tissues or canals, reducing the discharge of fluids.

atmosphere—Commonly used as a unit of pressure. "One atmosphere" is equal to 14.7 lbs/ft^2.

autoclave—A vessel capable of containing high pressure steam in which packaged pharmaceuticals are sterilized.

B

B$_2$O$_3$—Boric oxide.

bactericide—A substance that kills bacteria.

bacteriostat—A substance that is added to a drug formulation to control the growth of bacteria.

barrier—Used in this book only in the sense of a barrier to the permeation of gases.

base—A chemical compound which, when dissolved in water, dissociates to form a hydroxyl ion and raises its pH above 7 (see ALKALI). Usually a metal oxide or hydroxide.

bioavailability—The availability of an administered drug to the circulatory system.

blister package—A package consisting of a cavity thermoformed from a thermoplastic and a flat lid heat sealed thereon.

brick pack—A paper container which incorporates an aluminum foil barrier and plastic components that seal the aluminum foil to the paper and which enable the container to be hermetically closed by heat sealing.

BTU—British thermal unit. A unit of energy.

buccal cavity—The cavity formed by the cheek.

buffer, buffered—A buffer is a substance which, when dissolved in water, acts to resist changes in pH that would otherwise be caused by environmental factors (CO_2 in air, alkaline materials in glass containers, etc.). A buffered solution contains such a buffering agent.

C

CaO—Calcium oxide.

caplet—A tablet shaped like a capsule.

capsule—A transparent, hard or soft, water soluble shell containing a drug preparation.

carboxyl group—A group with the structure —COOH.

catalyst—A chemical compound that accelerates the rate of a chemical reaction without being consumed in the process.

caustic—A strong base, usually sodium hydroxide.

CFR—Code of Federal Regulations.

CGMP—Current Good Manufacturing Practice, often abbreviated GMP.

chipboard—A low-grade board made from wastepaper.

Class I recall—A drug recall in which there is a possibility that death could result if the drug was not recalled.

Class 100, Class 1000—Refers to work areas in which the air contains, per cubic foot, no more than 100 (or 1000) particles 0.5 microns in size or larger.

coefficient of thermal expansion—A dimensionless number that expresses the degree to which a material will expand when subjected to a known and specified increase in temperature.

coextrude—To simultaneously extrude more than one polymer layer.

colitis—Inflammation of the colon.

comonomer—One component of a copolymer, chemically distinct from the other comonomers.

compliance—Adherence by a patient to the drug regimen prescribed by the doctor.

controlled substance—A drug that is subject to the Controlled Substances Act of 1970 which sets limitations on its prescription and requirements for storage and record keeping depending on the potential for physical or psychological dependence.

copolymer—A polymer formed from at least two different comonomers.

corona treatment—Subjecting a polymer film to an electrical discharge to alter its surface characteristics.

cosmetic—Formulated products used to decorate, adorn or beautify but which have no therapeutic effect or purpose.

count—As in *100-count bottle*—the number of items (tablets, capsules) in the container; also used to specify that the container can hold this number of items.

CPSC—Consumer Product Safety Commission.

CRC—Child-resistant closure.

cream—A medicated preparation based on an emulsion of oil in water.

cross-link—To join separate polymer chains by means of short molecular fragments which bond to both chains.

CT—Continuous thread.

cul-de-sac—A sac-like cavity such as that formed between the eye and the eyelid.

D

deadfold—When a film, or any web, does not spring back after being folded, it is said to have "good deadfold." Most plastic films have poor deadfold compared to paper and metal foil.

deliquescent—Refers to a substance that readily absorbs moisture.

demulcent—A substance formulated to soothe the part of the body to which it is applied.

depyrogenation—The elimination of pyrogens by heat or a chemical process.

dermatological—Relating to diseases of the skin.

diacid—An organic acid containing two carboxyl groups.

dialysis—The process of separating mixed substances in solution by means of a membrane that is permeable only to some of the components and not to others.

dielectric heating—Creating heat in non-conductive substances, such as plastics, by subjecting them to a high-frequency electrical field which causes rapid molecular vibration.

diester—An organic molecule containing two ester groups.

dioxin—A complex organic compound that can form during incineration of organic materials that contain chlorine atoms. Toxic to animals and a cause of chloracne in humans.

dispersion coating—A coating process in which the coating material is suspended in the coating bath, as contrasted to solvent coating, in which the coating agent is dissolved in the bath.

distillation—The process in which a liquid is purified by transforming it into a vapor, separating the vapor from the impure liquid, and then condensing and collecting it.

diuretic—A drug formulation that increases urinary discharge.

DMF—Drug Master File.

dosage form—The form of a drug preparation that determines how the drug is administered: tablet, oral liquid, suppository, parenteral liquid, etc.

E

EAA—Ethylene acrylic acid.

effervescent—Refers to substances that produce a gas, usually carbon dioxide, upon mixing with water.

efficacy—The term used to describe the effectiveness of a drug in treating the condition it is designed to treat.

efflorescent—Refers to substances which lose water on exposure to air.

elastomer—A polymer with elastic characteristics similar to rubber—the ability to be stretched to at least twice its original length without sustaining permanent deformation.

elixirs—Syrups containing 20–25% alcohol.

emollients—Substances which soften and relax the tissues when applied locally.

emulsion—A liquid consisting of a discontinuous, immiscible liquid phase dispersed in a continuous liquid phase.

enteric—Refers to coatings which delay dissolution until a solid dosage form reaches the intestine.

EPDM—Elastomers based on terpolymers of ethylene, propylene, and a diene monomer such as 1,4-hexadiene.

epidermis—The first inner layer of the skin.

ester—The reaction product of an acid and an alcohol that contains a $-COO-$ group.

EVOH—Ethylene vinyl alcohol, a copolymer of ethylene and vinyl alcohol.

F

FDA—Food and Drug Administration.

filtration—The process by which solid particles are removed from a liquid by passing the liquid through a porous medium whose pores are so small that the solid particles will not pass through them.

finish—As applied to bottles and closures, describes the thread design: the size, pitch, profile, length, and thickness.

fluidized bed—A group of solid particles in a container that are agitated by an upward-flowing stream of gas.

fluorocarbon—An organic compound containing fluorine.

flux—A substance or mixture used to promote the fusion of metals or minerals. Often called a *fluxing agent*.

free radical—A highly reactive species formed by the rupture of a chemical bond.

fusion seal—A seal created by melting the adjacent surfaces that are to be sealed together.

G

gang printing—The practice of printing groups of several different labels consecutively on a single roll of labelstock.

gastrointestinal—The system of body organs that includes the stomach and small intestine.

g/cc—Grams per cubic centimeter.

gel—A colloidal semisolid consisting of a network structure of suspended, fine, solid particles surrounded by a liquid. Differs from a colloidal solution, which has no solid character, by having sufficient bonding between the solid particles to confer some rigidity to the structure.

gelatin—A water soluble substance extracted from animal tissue and bones and used in the manufacturing of capsules.

generic—Used in the pharmaceutical business to describe any drug that is labeled for sale with its technical name rather than a trade name (e.g., *diazepam* rather than *Valium*) and usually manufactured by companies that were not the original developer of the product.

glassine—A highly compacted grease-proof paper produced by calendering at very high pressure in the presence of steam.

GMP—Good Manufacturing Practice. *See* CGMP.

H

haze—A term used to characterize the milky appearance of a polymer film that is caused when light is scattered by surface imperfections or film inhomogeneities.

HDPE—High density polyethylene.

hermetic seal, hermetic container—Any seal, or any container so sealed, that is impervious to all gases under normal conditions of handling and storage.

HF—Hydrofluoric acid.

HIPS—High-impact polystyrene.

hologram—The image formed by a lensless photographic process (holography) that uses laser light to produce three-dimensional images.

hormone—A substance formed in and secreted by the endocrine glands. Often made synthetically.

hydrocarbon—An organic compound containing only carbon and hydrogen.

hydrolysis—Reaction of a compound with water resulting in destruction of the compound and the formation of at least two new ones.

hypoglycemia—An abnormally small concentration of glucose in the circulating blood.

I

IND—Investigational new drug.

induction heating—Heating a metal object by application of an external magnetic field to generate heat-producing eddy currents in the object.

infusion—Introduction of a fluid other than blood (e.g., saline solution) into a vein.

inhalant—A substance that can be vaporized by mechanical means or by heat and carried into the respiratory tract by inhalation.

innerseal—A membrane sealed across the top of a container to act as a barrier and as a tamper evident device.

intermediate—Used in manufacturing chemistry to denote a compound used in the manufacture of another.

intracisternal—Introduction of a cannula into the cisterna cerebellomedullaris for aspiration of cerebrospinal fluid or injection of air into the ventricles of the brain.

intravenous—Administration of a drug by injection directly into a vein.

in vitro—Refers to chemical or physical tests of drugs using laboratory procedures and apparatus.

in vivo—Refers to tests of drugs in animals or humans.

ion—A charged atom or group of atoms formed by the dissociation of a molecule, often in an aqueous medium.

ionomer—A copolymer containing acid groups, some of which are neutralized with metal ions such as sodium or zinc.

IR—Infrared.

irrigation—Washing out a cavity or wound with fluid.

isotonicity—The situation obtained when the colligative or osmotic properties of a pharmaceutical are matched with those of the biological site of administration, frequently mucous membranes.

IV—Intravenous.

K

kaolin—A family of clays containing combinations of hydrated alumina and silica.

keratolytic—A medication used to treat conditions that lead to horny skin growths.

kpsi—1000 psi.

L

labile—Free to move. In chemistry, used to characterize a molecule or group that readily moves within the molecular environment to link up with other molecules or with other species like itself.

lactose—A crystalline, sweet, water soluble disaccharide found in milk.

laminate—A multilayer web in which the layers are tightly adhered to one another by adhesives or by fusion bonding.

latex, latices—The milky juice or exudation of plants obtained by tapping the trunk, usually of a rubber tree.

LDPE—Low density polyethylene.

light resistant container—A container that protects the contents from the effects of light.

lipophilic—Having a strong affinity for oily or fatty substances.

LLDPE—Linear low density polyethylene.

lot, lot number—A *lot* refers to all the product made during a single run on a piece of equipment. A run may last for minutes, hours, or even days, but when it is stopped and the equipment or ingredients are altered to produce something else, the production of that lot is complete. A *lot number* is the number assigned to that lot.

lyophilization—Freeze-drying. The removal of water from a substance by applying a vacuum to the substance after it has been frozen.

M

m²—square meter.

magma, milk—Highly thickened suspensions for oral administration.

mandrel—A metal rod or bar used as a core around which metal, glass, etc., is cast, molded or shaped.

melt index—A measure of the viscosity of a polymer melt. The higher the melt index, the lower the viscosity.

melt viscosity—The viscosity of a molten polymer, i.e., its resistance to flow.

metallized—Possessing a submicron-thickness coating of a metal which has been applied by a vacuum process.

mg—milligram

microencapsulated—The encasement of small particles, either solid or liquid, within a shell that prevents their escape until the shell is ruptured by an external force or dissolved by a solvent.

micron—One ten-thousandth of a centimeter.

microorganisms, microbes—Living microscopic entities including bacteria and molds.

migration—When used in the drug packaging context, refers to the movement of substances through the wall of the package, a phenomenon which is often undesirable since the package contents may become adulterated by the migration of container components into said contents.

mil—One-thousandth of an inch.

modulus—A general expression, better particularized as *tensile modulus* or *elastic modulus*. Modulus is the slope of the line generated when stress is plotted against strain. A high slope (high modulus) characterizes a stiff material.

MnO_2—Manganese dioxide.

moisture permeability—The transmission of moisture through a membrane, film, or package. For a package, the rate of this process is expressed as milligrams per day per liter of container volume. *See* WVTR.

mucous membrane—The lining of the mouth, throat, and nasal and bronchial passages.

multiple dose container—A multiple unit container for parenteral formulations.

multiple unit container—One that permits withdrawal of part of the contents while containing and protecting the un-withdrawn balance.

N

Na_2O—Sodium oxide.

NDA—New Drug Application. Submitted to the FDA for each new drug or drug package.

NDC—National Drug Code.

NF—National Formulary.

O

ointment—A medicated preparation with an oleaginous base. More generally, any semisolid preparation intended for topical administration.

oleaginous base—A base with the nature or quality of an oil.

ophthalmic—Related to the eye.

OPP—Oriented polypropylene.

optical isomers—Isomers that have the same empirical and structural formula but which differ in the location of substituent groups around a central carbon atom. In their pure form, they rotate the plane of incident polarized light that is passed through them.

organosol—A colloidal dispersion of an organic solid in an organic solvent.

orient, oriented—The alignment of polymer molecules in a film.

OTC—Over-the-counter.

otic—Related to the ear.

outsert—Supplementary labeling information in the form of a printed leaflet adhered to the outside of a package with adhesive, or held in place by an overwrap.

overseal—In packaging, any device applied over the primary closure to hold it firmly in place and/or to supplement its gas barrier.

oxidation—Reaction with oxygen. More generally, removal of electrons from an atom or molecule.

P

parenteral—Describes any drug intended for administration by injection: subcutaneously, intramuscularly or intravenously.

parison—A partially formed bottle of glass or plastic which is subsequently formed by blowing into the finished shape.

partial pressure—When a mixture of gases is contained in a vessel, the pressure exerted on the vessel walls by just one of the gaseous species is known as the partial pressure of that species. The sum of all the partial pressures is equal to the total pressure exerted by the gas mixture.

PbO_2—Lead dioxide.

PE—Polyethylene.

peptide—Compound made up of two or more amino acids joined through an amide linkage.

perfluorinated—An organic compound that has all of its hydrogen atoms replaced by fluorine atoms.

peridural—Upon or outside the dura mater, a tough fibrous membrane forming the outer envelope of the brain.

permeation—The movement of a labile substance, usually a gas, through a solid by diffusion. In packaging, used to describe the movement of gases through the package walls.

PET—Polyethylene terephthalate.

petrolatum—A gelatinous or oily translucent substance obtained from petroleum.

pH—A measure of the hydrogen ion concentration in, and the acidity of, an aqueous solution.

pharmaceutical—A manufactured, processed or compounded form of a drug.

plasticizer—A substance mixed into a plastic to decrease its stiffness and increase its softness.

plastisol—A plastic used in the form of an emulsion, e.g., for coating.

polyglycols—Polymers made from glycols, which are organic molecules containing at least two hydroxyl (OH) groups.

polymer—A high molecular weight molecule formed by reacting small molecules (monomers) together to form a long chain consisting of many monomer units.

polyolefin—Any polymer whose monomer units are unsaturated hydrocarbons (olefins) containing only carbon and hydrogen. Polyethylene and polypropylene are the most common polyolefins used in packaging.

PP—Polypropylene.

ppb—Parts per billion.

primary package—The package that contains the product being packaged.

prophylaxis—Prevention of disease or its spread by the administration of drugs and/or other procedures.

protein—Complex organic compounds containing amino acids essential to tissue growth and repair.

protocol—A set of procedures. *Test protocols*, for example, are the set of instructions that govern how a test is run.

PS—Polystyrene.

PTFE—Polytetrafluoroethylene.

pulpboard—See CHIPBOARD.

PVC—Polyvinyl chloride.

PVDC—Polyvinylidene chloride.

pyrogen—Agent that causes a rise in body temperature, especially if injected. The most important pyrogen in sterile drug manufacture is endotoxin, a residue from gram-negative bacteria.

R

racemization—The conversion of a dextro (*d*) or levo (*l*) optical isomer into an equilibrium mixture of the two.

rectal mucosa—The outer layer of the lining of the rectum.

resin—The term for a polymer in the form of small pellets that is packaged in a bag or in bulk and shipped to a processor.

respiratory system—The body system that includes the mouth, nose, throat, bronchial passages and lungs.

reverse osmosis—The process in which the solute in a solution is removed by forcing the solvent, against the normal osmotic pressure, to flow through a membrane that is not permeable to the solute. Widely used to remove salts from seawater.

RH—Relative humidity.

roll stock—A web wound up on a roll and fed therefrom to a process such as printing, wrapping or labeling.

S

saturated—When used to describe a type of chemical bond or molecule, the bonding is saturated if no double or triple bonds exist, i.e., each atom is joined within the molecule to other atoms only by single bonds.

scabacide—A substance which destroys the organism causing scabies.

secondary package—The package that contains the primary package. Usually a box.

semipermeable membrane—A membrane that permits the passage of one or more components of a solution but does not allow the passage of other components. Such membranes are usually permeable only to the solvent.

shelf life—The time required for the potency of a drug to drop to 90% of its labeled potency.

silicone—Polymers composed of molecular chains containing alternating silicon and oxygen atoms. These can be liquids or solids depending on the molecular weight and the groups attached to the chain.

single dose container—A single unit container for parenterals only.

single unit container—A container that holds the quantity of drug intended for administration as a single dose promptly after the container is opened.

SiO_2—Silicon dioxide (silica).

SO_2—Sulfur dioxide.

Sol—A colloidal solution or the liquid phase of a colloidal solution.

solvent coating—Coating a web (plastic, paper, etc.) with materials by passing the web through a solution of the coating materials and then evaporating the solvent from the layer of liquid that remains on the web. Differs from *dispersion coating* (see DISPERSION COATING) in that in the latter process, the coating components are suspended, rather than dissolved, in the coating bath.

sorb, sorption—In drug packaging, the removal of pharmaceutical components by a package by adsorption onto the package surface or absorption onto the package wall.

stearate—A waxy salt of stearic acid derived from animal fat.

sterile, sterility—The absence of microorganisms.

steroid—Fat-soluble organic compounds such as sterols, bile acids, and sex hormones.

stratum corneum—The outermost layer of the skin.

strength—In pharmaceutical parlance, the amount of active ingredient in a preparation.

stress crack—The solvent-induced generation of cracks in a plastic object. Typically occurs in areas of unrelieved stress.

strip package—A package made by enclosing an object to be packaged, such as a tablet, between two webs and then sealing the webs together so that the seal completely surrounds the object being packaged.

subcutaneous—Beneath the skin.

sublingual—Under the tongue.

substrate—In packaging, refers to a surface, normally a web, onto which is applied other materials designed to alter the characteristics or properties of the original web.

suppository—The dosage form designed for insertion into the rectum.

surfactant—Any substance, but normally a soap or a detergent, that forms a compatibilizing boundary layer between two liquids or a liquid and a solid. This layer leads to the stable dispersion of one phase in another—a liquid in another liquid or a solid in a liquid.

suspension—Solid particles dispersed in a liquid. If the suspension is stable, it will resist the normal gravitational separation into two phases.

systemic—Administration of a drug so that it gains access to the circulatory system.

T

tablet triturate—A tablet that dissolves readily in the mouth.

tack, tacky—The tendency for a material to stick to itself and other objects. Stickiness, sticky.

talc—A naturally occurring white mineral containing hydrated magnesium oxide and silica.

tensile modulus—See MODULUS.

tensile strength—The resistance of a specimen to breaking when stressed longitudinally.

tertiary package—The package that holds the secondary package. Usually a corrugated shipping container.

therapeutic—Relating to the treatment of disease.

thermoform—To form a plastic sheet into a shape by using pressure to force the heat-softened plastic into a mold.

thermoplastic—Describes any substance that becomes more pliable as it is heated. In packaging, used to denote that class of plastics which can be formed when hot but become stiff after cooling.

thermoset—The class of plastics which become rigid when heated. The opposite of thermoplastics, which become pliable when heated.

tight container—A container that protects its contents from contamination by extraneous liquids, solids, or gases; from physical loss of the drug and from efflorescence, deliquescence, or evaporation under the ordinary or customary conditions of handling, shipment, storage, and distribution. See Chapter Eight for quantitative definition. See *also* WELL-CLOSED CONTAINER.

TiO$_2$—Titanium dioxide.

tincture—A solution of a drug in alcohol.

topical—Administration of a drug to the skin surface or the lining of body cavities. The therapeutic purpose is usually limited to localized areas.

toxin—A noxious or poisonous substance formed during the growth of certain microorganisms.

toxoid—A toxin that has been treated, e.g., with formaldehyde, to destroy its toxic property but retain its antigenicity, i.e., its capability of stimulating the production of antitoxin antibodies and thus providing immunity.

transdermal—Administration of drugs through the skin.

Type I glass—Glass composed largely of silica and boric oxide that is very low in water-extractible impurities.

Type II glass—Glass containing larger amounts of water-soluble sodium and calcium oxides than are present in Type I glass.

Type III glass—Glass containing even greater quantities of water-extractable oxides than Type II glass.

U

unit dose container—A single unit container for articles intended for administration by other than the parenteral route as a single dose, direct from the container.

unsaturated—When used in discussing molecules or chemical bonding, this term characterizes molecules that contain multiple bonds, i.e., some of the atoms are joined to others by more than one bond.

unsupported—An unsupported film is not bonded to another film or substrate that would give it mechanical support. Used most frequently to denote aluminum foil that is not bonded to any other material, web or substrate.

urethra—The tube that drains the bladder to the outside of the body.

USP—United States Pharmacopoeia. See Chapter Three for a detailed definition. When in italics, *USP* refers to the Compendium published by USP.

UV—Ultraviolet.

V

validation—Testing the components of an operation to confirm that they are performing the function they are supposed to perform. See Chapter Seven for a more elaborate definition.

vasoconstrictors—Drugs that reduce the flow of body fluids by constricting the ducts, tubes, and canals through which these fluids flow.

vasodilators—Drugs that increase the flow of body fluids by relaxing the muscles surrounding the ducts, tubes, and canals through which those fluids flow.

vinyl—A common term for polyvinyl chloride.

W

wavelength—The distance between identical points in a wave pattern. A measure of the energy content of light—the shorter the wavelength, the higher the energy level.

web—In packaging, a term that denotes a plastic film or a length of paper that is either part of or is being drawn off a large roll for processing, e.g., for coating or for wrapping an object. For example, a *printed web* would be a roll of printed film; *apply the adhesive to the web* would mean applying the adhesive to the film as it is being unwound from the roll.

well-closed container—A container that protects its contents from extraneous solids and from physical loss of the contents under the ordinary and customary conditions of handling, shipment, and distribution. See TIGHT CONTAINER and Chapter Eight for a quantitative description.

WVTR—Water vapor transmission rate.

INDEX